$\mathcal{S}$ TRAIGHT TALK *about* BREAST CANCER

FROM DIAGNOSIS TO RECOVERY

Sixth Edition

SUZANNE W. BRADDOCK, M.D.
JANE M. KERCHER, M.D.
JOHN J. EDNEY, M.D.
MARGARET BLOCK, M.D.
MELANIE MORRISSEY CLARK

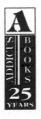

Addicus Books
Omaha, Nebraska

An Addicus Nonfiction Book

ISBN 978-1-943886-81-4
Cover design by Peri Poloni-Gabriel
Typography and illustrations by Jack Kusler

This book is not intended to be a substitute for a physician, nor do the authors intend to give advice contrary to that of an attending physician.

All proceeds from the sale of this book are donated to the *Straight Talk about Breast Cancer Charitable Trust* and are used to assist breast cancer patients and their families.

Library of Congress Cataloging-in-Publication Data

Names: Braddock, Suzanne W., – author. | Kercher, Jane M., author. | Edney, John J., author. | Block, Margaret, author. | Clark, Melanie Morrissey, author.
Title: Straight talk about breast cancer : from diagnosis to recovery / Suzanne Braddock, M.D., Jane Kercher, M.D., John J. Edney, M.D., Margaret Block, M.D., Melanie Morrissey Clark.
Description: Sixth edition. | Omaha, Nebraska : Addicus Books, Inc., [2019] | "An Addicus Nonfiction Book." | Includes bibliographical references and index.
Identifiers: LCCN 2019019816 (print) | LCCN 2019020121 (ebook) | ISBN 9781950091164 (pdf) | ISBN 9781950091188 (kdl) | ISBN 9781950091171 (epub)
Subjects: LCSH: Breast—Cancer—Popular works.
Classification: LCC RC280.B8 (ebook) | LCC RC280.B8 S748 2019 (print) | DDC 616.99/449—dc23
LC record available at https://lccn.loc.gov/2019019816

Addicus Books, Inc.
P.O. Box 45327
Omaha, Nebraska 68145
AddicusBooks.com
Printed in the United States of America
10 9 8 7 6 5 4 3 2 1

To all women with breast cancer
and to their families

CONTENTS

Preface

Please read this book imagining that a very good friend is sitting close to you, giving you an introduction to the rest of your life with love and understanding. Imagine your friend—who has indeed walked in your shoes—taking you by the hand and guiding you through the next few weeks.

Your friend wants to help you understand what is happening, and help you cope with the decisions and treatments ahead. She also wants to help your family and friends, for they are suffering with you.

Know there will come a time when you'll go entire minutes without thinking of breast cancer—then hours, and even days. Of course, your life will never be the same. In fact, it will probably be better in many ways you would not have chosen but will be delighted to discover.

The authors of this book, now in its sixth edition, reach out to you as dear friends and offer you the hope of a complete recovery, along with the certainty that your journey from here will be one of growth, challenge, and change. That is, after all, what life is about.

ACKNOWLEDGMENTS

W e, the authors, would like to thank those who helped make this book possible. We are grateful to physicians Robert Langdon Jr., M.D., Patrick McKenna, M.D., Janalyn Prows, M.D., the late Henry Lynch, M.D., Ramon Fusaro, M.D., John J. Heieck, M.D., Richard Bruneteau, M.D., Carol Kornhehl, M.D., author of *The Best News about Radiation Therapy,* and Karen Sublett, R.N., Clinical Nurse Specialist, Oncology.

We thank Mollie Foster, Ph.D., for her contributions and Judy Dierkhising, Ph.D., for her insights into the emotional needs of breast cancer patients. Our appreciation goes to the Nebraska Methodist Hospital Breast Cancer Support Group for their comments, wit, and strength. And with gratitude, we remember Sue Kocsis, a real spark, whose encouragement meant so much during the early stages of this book. We thank Chris Hinz for her contributions to the metastatic breast cancer chapter.

We are also deeply grateful to the women who shared their personal stories in order to help others. A special thanks to the women who shared their surgery and reconstruction photos. We acknowledge photographers Larry Ferguson and Paula Friedland for their creativity and sensitivity in portraying these women as real, living people, rather than medical subjects. We thank Jack Kusler, of Addicus Books, who provided illustrations and designed the layout of the book. We are also indebted to our publisher of twenty-five years, Rod Colvin for his encouragement and support.

Introduction

Someone you love or someone you know will get breast cancer—your friend, your aunt, your mother, your father, your daughter, yourself. The fact is, if you are an American woman, your chance of getting breast cancer is especially high—about one in eight over your lifetime. The chance of dying from breast cancer is one in thirty-six. Each year in the United States, approximately 270,000 women are diagnosed with breast cancer.

Here's the good news: Thanks to early detection and better ways to treat breast cancer, more and more women with breast cancer are surviving. The percentage has climbed steadily since 1989—not just five-year disease-free survival, either, but real, lasting, bounce-the-grandkids-on-your-knee survival.

The rest of my life started April 1, 1992, with a phone call from my friend and doctor, who informed me that the lump in my breast was malignant. I reacted, as do most women, with the irrational certainty that I was going to die, and soon. I was forty-nine.

Fortunately, my cancer had not yet spread when it was diagnosed, at least not that the existing technology could determine. The tumor was medium-size—2.2 centimeters, a little under an inch in diameter.

Surgery is almost always recommended for breast cancer. I chose to have a mastectomy—surgery to remove the breast—followed by chemotherapy. Women with breast cancer are offered chemotherapy when their tumors are of a certain size or if they are in a high-risk category for recurrence. Follow-up treatments such as chemotherapy and other drugs can prevent or postpone a recurrence of the cancer and improve the chance of long-term survival.

The usual chemotherapy for early-stage breast cancer, although no picnic, is no longer the ordeal it used to be. Now there are drugs to help with nausea and fatigue, and to stimulate blood-cell production in the bone marrow—thereby helping to prevent infection and possibly detrimental treatment delays.

Of course, chemotherapy has turned wig making into a real growth industry. My daughter, Gail, had a lot of fun playing with my wig—or, as we called it, "the muskrat." Actually, I learned to appreciate the ease with which I could wash my "hair"—swish it in a bowl of suds, rinse it, and hang it to dry. I also enjoyed snatching it off at stoplights on the hot drive home from work and chuckling at other drivers' startled expressions.

Going through surgery and chemotherapy mobilized me, and it was easy to focus on milestones: one-third done, halfway done—finished! My eyelashes returned, and before I knew it, I was ready to donate the muskrat to the American Cancer Society's wig bank. I could climb the hill behind my house without gasping for breath, and, finally, I went an entire day without thinking about breast cancer.

My days now, after breast cancer, are as precious as the glimpse of a small garden behind a city brownstone. These are good days. They have shown me, in a poignant and powerful way, that life is best lived by us all, with or without cancer, in a state of radical trust. Trust, and trust, and trust some more. None of us knows the limits of our days, but we do know Who limits them. And that is all we need to know.

—*Suzanne W. Braddock, M.D.*

Wind

I sit silent in the cold room, reading,
when softly, a stir outside calls me away. It is the wind,
moving the frozen oaks and evergreens, pushing the
snow across the ice on the lake.
It is a sound both great and small,
the breath of God over the land,
the voice of creation,
giving life to this cold, barren landscape,
to my days of terror.
I feel the power embraced in that sound,
and joy in the force that is greater than I,
greater than cancer,
greater than all the pain in all the women.

—*Suzanne W. Braddock, M.D.*

1

BREAST CANCER:
AN OVERVIEW

A diagnosis of breast cancer is never good news. However, research continues at a brisk pace in breast cancer prevention, diagnosis, and treatment, and the research has produced positive results. Since 1989, the death rate from this disease has declined by approximately 40 percent, even though the number of cases has gradually risen. Approximately 270,000 women are diagnosed with breast cancer each year in the United States. The majority of women whose breast cancer is discovered early are cured.

Partly because of a surge in breast cancer awareness, more and more women are learning about this illness and about their own level of risk. The more they know, the more faithfully they practice self-examination, schedule mammograms, and take care of their health. In turn, more cases of breast cancer are detected early and the survival rate continues to rise.

You can see why every woman, regardless of her age, needs information about breast cancer—especially in the United States, where the breast cancer rate is among the highest in the world. If you have breast cancer, knowledge is the most potent antidote to fear and the best preparation for treatment. If you do not have breast cancer, knowledge is your strongest protection.

The best way to start learning about breast cancer is with an understanding of the healthy breast.

Breast Anatomy

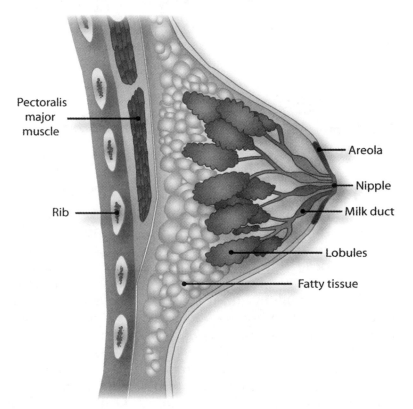

Pectoralis major muscle

Rib

Areola

Nipple

Milk duct

Lobules

Fatty tissue

Breast Structure and Function

The human female breast is so glamorized and commercialized in our culture, it's easy to forget that the breast has a serious job—producing milk for babies. Even a quick look at breast structure reminds us of this important function.

The breast is made up of fatty tissue that contains blood vessels and lymph vessels, plus fifteen to twenty rounded divisions called *lobes,* themselves formed of dozens of smaller *lobules* that end in tiny *bulbs.* The lobular system produces milk in response to hormonal changes after childbirth or after an abortion or a late miscarriage.

Milk flows from the lobes and bulbs through narrow tubes, or *ducts,* leading to the *nipple,* which protrudes from the center of the *areola*—the circle of darker skin at the tip of the breast.

Lymph vessels in the breast carry *lymph,* a pale fluid containing white blood cells, to *lymph nodes*—small, rounded masses of tissue that act as filters for this fluid. Lymph serves to transport infection-fighting cells to all parts of the body. There are lymph vessels and nodes throughout the body, but the lymph nodes nearest to the breast are *usually* the first ones affected when breast cancer begins to spread.

Breast cancer is not a death sentence. We've made so much progress in the last twenty years. In the future, I believe breast cancer will be viewed more as a chronic disease, like hypertension or diabetes.

—Kathryn, oncology RN

How Cancer Develops

Every part of your body, and of every other living thing, is made up of cells. In human beings, some cells divide to create new cells every twelve to twenty-four hours. In the normal, orderly cell-renewal process, cells reproduce just fast enough to replace the ones that die off, keeping your blood and organs healthy.

Cancer forms when cells become abnormal and start to divide uncontrollably. Eventually, an abnormal growth, or *tumor,* may form. Tumor cells not only act differently from normal cells, but they also look different under a microscope.

Some tumors are *benign*—not cancerous. Benign tumors do not spread, so surgically removing them usually solves the problem. By contrast, a *malignant* (cancerous) tumor—if not detected and treated early—may spread from its original site to other parts of the body in a process called *metastasis*. Malignant tumors may be removed by surgery and treated with one or more additional types of therapy, depending on how large they are and whether they have metastasized.

Most breast cancers develop in the lobes or ducts of the breast. Scientists are still learning exactly how this occurs; they have identified certain risk factors—some proven, others more questionable. It is helpful to be aware of all risk factors.

I don't care how many breasts my mom has. I'm just happy she's okay.

—*Gail, 13*

Risk Factors for Breast Cancer

Age

A woman's risk of developing this disease increases as she gets older—80 percent of breast cancers in women are diagnosed after the age of fifty. Even though aging is a risk factor, you can be proactive by getting regular mammograms and staying healthy to minimize risk factors.

Environmental Risks

Every day, we are exposed to toxins in the form of pesticides, herbicides, cleaning solvents, chemical waste, food additives, certain plastics, and many other substances. Some are known *carcinogens* (cancer-causing agents). Others have been linked to higher rates of cancer among people exposed to them, but the cause has not been scientifically proven.

Hormonal Risks

Compared to the general population, a woman is at greater risk for breast cancer if she has been exposed to higher levels of estrogen over her lifetime. This exposure can be entirely natural, due to the following factors:

- early onset of menstrual periods (before age 12)
- late menopause (after age 55)
- late first pregnancy (after age 30)
- no pregnancies

Also contributing to lifetime estrogen exposure are medicines that contain estrogen, such as birth control pills and drugs taken to ease menopausal symptoms. Most researchers doubt that the synthetic hormones in birth control pills pose much of a breast cancer risk. Some studies suggest a slightly higher risk among long-term users of oral contraception and among women who started using them as teenagers.

Long-term estrogen-replacement therapy, during and after menopause, is a risk factor that diminishes when use of the hormone is stopped. Certain hormone combinations, however, are more carcinogenic than treatment with estrogen alone. One of these combinations is estrogen and progesterone, which is sold under several brand names. If you're taking a prescription drug for menopause symptoms, ask your doctor if it contains one of these combinations and, if so, whether you should switch to another drug.

Radiation Exposure

Women who have had radiation to the chest—perhaps as treatment for cancers such as Hodgkin's disease or for conditions such as tuberculosis or breast inflammation (mastitis)—are at greater risk for breast cancer.

If you have been treated with radiation to the chest, you should begin regular breast self-examination and annual mammograms no later than ten years after the radiation treatment began. These precautions are all the more important if you were exposed during puberty, since developing breasts are especially vulnerable. You should also consider yearly MRI of your breasts.

The small amount of radiation delivered in chest X-rays and mammograms is not a cause for concern—

except possibly for women who have inherited mutated BRCA1 or BRCA2 genes.

These genes are intended to repair cell tissues; however, if they become damaged, their malfunction may result in the formation of breast cancer.

Diet and Drinking Alcohol

If you are overweight, especially if you put on those excess pounds during adulthood, your risk is higher than other women's. The same is true if you drink alcohol. The more you drink and the younger you start, the higher the risk. As little as three alcoholic drinks a week increases the risk for women.

After my diagnosis, I dealt with anxiety by saying, "I'm alive today and will live today to the hilt." By fearing death, I figured I was dying all the time instead of living.

—Suzanne, 58

Nationality and Ethnicity

North America has one of the highest incidences of breast cancer in the world, followed by Western Europe, Australia/New Zealand, and Northern Europe. The incidence is lowest in China and Central Africa. Genetic factors play a part, but environment and lifestyle may be equally important, since second- and third-generation immigrants to the United States are more likely to get breast cancer than their nonimmigrant relatives.

In the United States, white women are at slightly greater risk for breast cancer than African American women, but the death rate is higher among African Americans. The risk is lower among Native American, Hispanic, and Asian women.

> ## Breast Cancer in Men
> Although it is rare, breast cancer does occur in men. According to the American Cancer Society, approximately 2,700 men between ages sixty and seventy are diagnosed annually. The odds of a man getting breast cancer in his lifetime is 1 in 1,000. The average age at diagnosis is 72. Symptoms include: a lump in the breast, nipple pain, inverted nipple, nipple discharge, sores on the nipple, and enlarged lymph nodes under the arm. Treatment for men is similar to that for women.

Family History

Women in Western industrial countries have a higher risk of breast cancer even if they do not have a family history of breast cancer. In fact, about 85 percent of breast cancer cases occur in women who do not have a family history of the disease. In the other 15 percent of cases, at least one relative—more often an aunt or a grandmother than a mother or a sister—has had breast cancer. When this family history exists, the disease may be referred to as *polygenic breast cancer.* Even with a family history of polygenic breast cancer, many family members do not develop the disease.

In about 8 percent of all breast cancers, the disease is clearly passed from generation to generation. The most-commonly mutated genes are *BRCA1* (pronounced BRACK-uh one) and *BRCA2*. BRCA is an abbreviation for "breast cancer." Every man and woman has two of each of these genes. The job of these two genes is to repair DNA damage, which can prevent disease such as cancer; however, sometimes these genes undergo structural changes, called *mutations,* which limit the cell's ability to repair DNA damage. As a result, the risk of breast cancer is increased. These gene mutations are responsible for *hereditary* breast cancer.

A father or mother with one mutated gene, whether or not he or she develops cancer, has a 50 percent chance of passing the mutation to the next generation. Accordingly, a woman can have hereditary breast cancer even though her mother and sisters stay cancer-free.

Approximately 55 to 65 percent of women who inherit a BRCA1 mutation will develop breast cancer by age seventy. About 39 percent of women with this mutation will develop ovarian cancer by age seventy. At the same time, 45 percent of women who inherit a BRCA2 mutation will develop breast cancer by age seventy, and 11 to 17 percent will develop ovarian cancer by age seventy.

Cancer research also shows that another gene, called *PALB2,* raises the risk of breast cancer in women nearly as much as the mutations in the BRCA1 and BRCA2 genes. Like the BRCA1 and BRCA2 genes, everyone has two pairs of the PALB2. It, too, is supposed to repair cell damage; however, this gene can also become mutated. Scientists found that women with the mutation *and* a strong family history of breast cancer had a 58 percent risk of developing the disease by age seventy. Those who had no family history of breast cancer, but who had a mutation of the PALB2 gene, had a 33 percent chance of developing a malignancy by age seventy.

Maintaining a positive attitude is very important as you go through the treatment. It may be the best medicine there is during breast cancer treatment.

—Ann, 53

Testing for Genetic Factors

If you have a family history of breast cancer, talk to your doctor about genetic testing to assess your risk of developing breast cancer or other cancers. Most insurance plans, including Medicare, usually pay for genetic testing. It takes about three weeks to receive test results for gene testing, but this information is helpful to both you and your physician in making decisions about breast surgery. The test can be expedited if necessary.

Genetic testing analyzes small samples of blood or saliva to determine whether you carry genes for inherited diseases. The results can help with cancer prevention; or, if you have cancer, the testing can help determine the best treatment.

2

Getting a Diagnosis

You may tell yourself, "It's probably nothing"— that lump or thickness you think you feel in your breast. Perhaps you're thinking you should wait a while before going to see your doctor. Maybe you're thinking it really isn't a lump and that it will go away. But now is not the time to listen to this inner voice.

It is important to investigate any suspicious change in your breast and schedule that mammogram and annual physical. Breast cancer tumors that can be felt are usually discovered by you or by your doctor during a routine physical. Most lumps that can't be felt show up in mammograms.

If you find a lump, the next step is to get a *diagnosis*— to find out whether it is caused by cancer or something else. Odds are, it's something else. Only about one out of five breast lumps is cancerous.

Methods of Examining the Breasts

Breast Self-Examination

Many women discover their own cancers during a *breast self-examination (BSE)*. That's why every woman should examine her breasts every month. BSE should become routine as soon as the breasts develop, or by age twenty at the latest.

Possible Warning Signs of Breast Cancer

During self-exams, watch for the following:

- a lump or thickening in the breast, surrounding area, or armpit
- swelling, redness, or rash
- puckering or dimpling of the skin
- skin texture like that of an orange (a condition called *peau d'orange*)
- itchiness, soreness, or scaling of the nipple
- drawing-in (retraction) of the nipple or another part of the breast
- unusual warmth that feels feverish in or near the breast
- any change in breast size, shape, or symmetry
- unusual pain in a part of the breast, armpit, or surrounding area
- bloody discharge from the nipple

Because the breasts tend to swell during the menstrual period, premenopausal women should perform BSE three to five days after their period ends. Postmenopausal women should examine their breasts on the same day every month, so that the date itself is a reminder.

Some women, especially those in high-risk categories, avoid BSE because they are afraid of what they might find. This avoidance is understandable. It's also unhealthy, emotionally and physically. Frequent, habitual self-examination is by far the best way to discover a cancer while it is small and highly treatable, and finding a small tumor is much better than finding a large one.

One excuse some women use for not doing BSE is that their breasts are always lumpy—the result of benign masses called *cysts* or *fibrocystic changes*. This condition is noncancerous.

If you have benign masses in your breasts, you might assume that you wouldn't notice a new lump or one that is unusual. But if you examine your breasts regularly, you'll learn the "terrain." After you're familiar with the

Breast Self-Exam (BSE)

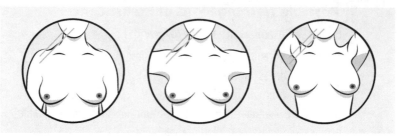

In front of a mirror, check for symmetry, nipple direction, and general appearance. Look for puckering, dimpling, skin changes, or dimpling.

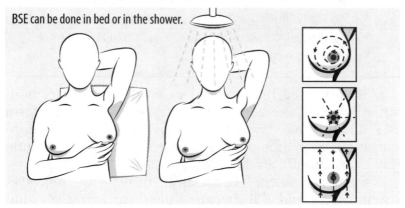

BSE can be done in bed or in the shower.

Examine the breast using light, firm pressure. Move fingers in dime-sized circles in the patterns shown on the right.

texture and the pattern of cysts in your breasts, you will be able to detect changes, even small ones.

Every month, use both BSE techniques described below: one lying down and one standing before a mirror.

Self-Examination Lying Down

To examine your breasts while lying down:

1. Place a small pillow under your right shoulder; then raise your right arm, and rest the back of your hand on your forehead. This position flattens the breast and makes it easier to examine.

2. Using the pads of the three middle fingers of your left hand, make small circular motions to examine

your right breast with light, medium, and then firm pressure. Don't lift your fingers but keep them flat as you do this.

3. Use an up-and-down pattern, as if following narrow vertical stripes, to cover the entire breast and surrounding area—from collarbone to lower bra line to breastbone, and including the armpit.

4. Repeat steps 1 through 3 using the right hand to examine the left breast.

5. You can examine your breasts this way in the shower or bathtub, although if you're not lying down you lose the advantage of your breasts being flattened, which makes abnormalities easier to find. On the other hand, slick, soapy skin makes small changes more noticeable. You can get the soapy-skin effect while lying down by applying a smooth lotion or placing a piece of slippery fabric (such as satin) over your breast while you examine it.

My diagnosis was unbelievable to me. The radiologist kept saying she was concerned about my mammogram and I kept saying it was just scar tissue from a previous biopsy. Then it dawned on me that she was trying to tell me she thought I had breast cancer.

—Ann, 53

Self-Examination Standing in Front of Mirror

To examine your breasts in front of a mirror, look for any of the warning signs listed above. Do this in each of the following positions:

- with your arms down at your sides
- with both arms held straight up over your head
- with your hands pressed against your hips to tighten the chest muscles and bending forward at the waist

If you notice a warning sign during BSE, or at any other time, see your doctor. Don't put it off, and if the doctor's office staff tries to schedule your visit for "the next available appointment" six months from now, ask to speak with the doctor's nurse or with the doctor.

Do not assume that a lump can't be cancer if it moves (or doesn't move) or if it is hard (or soft), tender (or painless), or regular (or irregular) in shape. Any new lump or thickening should be examined by a doctor, regardless of its characteristics.

It is never safe to stop doing BSE. It should be a lifelong habit, even if you have had a mastectomy (surgical removal of the breast) or lumpectomy (removal only of the tumor and a surrounding margin of healthy tissue to be examined for cancer cells). After surgery, begin examining the incision right away for changes, bumps, rigid areas, or discoloration, and search for lumps above and below the collarbone and in the armpit. Practicing BSE on the other breast is extremely important, too. Survivors of some types of breast cancer are at high risk for a new breast cancer in the opposite breast.

When I was diagnosed, tears came to my eyes, but I was more worried about my husband and two boys. How would they handle it if something happened to me? My main thought was helping them get through this.

—*Julianne, 54*

Clinical Examination

In addition to doing your own breast self-exams, you should always have a clinical breast exam as part of your annual checkup. In this exam, your doctor will feel the breasts and breast area for thickening or lumps, check for visible warning signs, and ask about breast tenderness or changes you might have experienced, your breast care, your medical history, and your family's medical history.

Mammogram

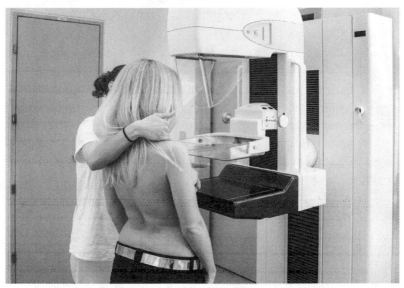

It's recommended that women have their first mammogram between the ages thirty-five at age forty. If you have a family history of breast cancer, talk to your doctor about a mammogram earlier.

Even though an experienced medical professional is usually more skilled than a patient at feeling the difference between a benign lump and a malignant one, he or she can't be certain whether a lump or another symptom indicates cancer. If the clinical exam raises suspicions of cancer, further diagnostic tests will be needed. The most common ones are described below.

Mammography

You've probably read or heard about the public debate over how soon a woman should begin having routine mammograms and whether or not mammograms are necessary for women in their forties. Please take note: The answer is: Yes they are! Mammograms save lives.

A *mammogram* is an X-ray of the breast. This test is simple, widely available, and lifesaving. Because of

---

Breast Cancer Screening Guidelines

The following guidelines for breast cancer screening are recommended by the American Cancer Society.

- Women ages 40 to 44 should have the choice to start annual mammograms.
- Women ages 45 to 54 should get annual mammograms.
- Women 55 and older should switch to mammograms every two years or can continue annual screening.

Screening should continue as long as a woman is in good health and is expected to live ten years or longer. Women with a family history of breast cancer should talk to their doctor about earlier screening.

---

mammograms, the number of deaths from breast cancer has fallen by nearly 40 percent since 1989.

Having a mammogram takes only a few minutes. It's simply a matter of standing next to a mammography machine while a technician positions your breast on a small, square plate, compresses it against another plate, and takes the image. The process is repeated—two images for each breast—and all you feel is a brief pinch during the short time your breast is positioned between the plates.

The images are captured either on film, like a photographic negative, or on solid-state detectors similar to those in digital cameras. In the latter case, the image is called a *digital mammogram.* Digital mammography exposes the breast to even less radiation than a film mammogram, produces more detailed images, and more accurately depicts the comparatively dense breasts of younger women. *Dense breast tissue* refers to the appearance of breast tissue on a mammogram. Women with dense breasts have more dense tissue than fatty tissue; density refers to milk glands, milk ducts, and supportive tissue. Whichever type of mammogram you have, a radiologist will interpret the images and you'll learn the results in a few days. Ideally, the same radiologist

3-D Mammography

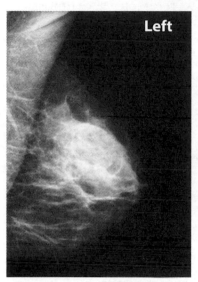
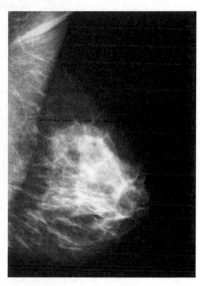

3-D mammograms provide a better view of breast tissues. Key studies show that 3-D mammograms have increased the detection of invasive cancers by approximately 40 percent and all breast cancers by 34 percent.

will read all your mammograms and compare your most recent images with your older ones.

Mammograms are done for either screening or diagnostic purposes. A *screening mammogram* searches for early cancers that cannot be felt; a diagnostic mammogram inspects a breast lump that can be felt or an abnormality detected in a screening mammogram. If you or your doctor finds a lump in your breast, a diagnostic mammogram is usually the next step.

A newer technology, known as a *3-D mammogram,* is a screening test that allows doctors to examine breast tissue more thoroughly. Also referred to as digital breast *tomosynthesis,* it creates three-dimensional pictures of the breast with X-rays.

Research shows that the 3-D mammogram, along with traditional digital mammography, detects up to 40 percent more invasive cancers and decreases false-positive rates by 15 percent. A *false positive* refers to a diagnosis of cancer when there is none.

If your breasts are healthy as far as you know, ask your doctor when to start having regular screening mammograms and how often you should have them. If you're in a high-risk category, your physician may want you to have your first mammogram while you're still in your twenties.

It is recommended that you seek out a certified breast center or clinic that offers digital mammography. By going to a certified facility, you can be assured that quality control measures are in place.

Waiting for test results, for information, is the hardest. When you're afraid, any wait at all seems too long.

—Ann, 53

If you have a family history of breast cancer, an annual mammogram starting when you are ten years younger than the earliest-diagnosed relative. For example, if your mother developed breast cancer at forty-five and your sister at thirty-two, you should start having annual mammograms at twenty-two.

Don't be alarmed if your mammogram shows abnormalities and your doctor wants to do additional tests. Only 5 to 10 percent of "suspicious" abnormalities turn out to be breast cancer. False-positive results are so common that most women who have regular mammograms will eventually get that dreaded phone call or letter asking them to return for further tests, only to find that there is nothing wrong.

Be grateful for false positives, and for your doctor's diligence in following up on a suspicious abnormality that turns out to be harmless. The inconvenience and expense of follow-up diagnostic studies (usually another mammogram or an ultrasound) are easily outweighed by the many lives mammography saves.

Sample Mammograms

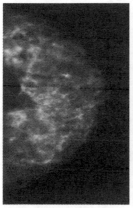

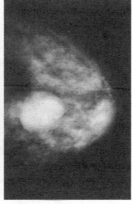

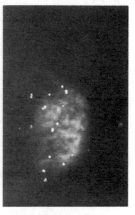

A normal mammogram

Mammogram showing cysts with smooth edges

Mammogram with benign calcifications scattered throughout

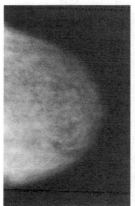

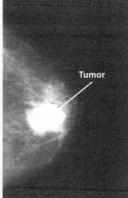

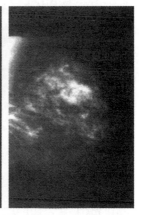

Mammogram showing a dense pattern, usually seen in younger women

Mammogram showing cancerous growth. Note the irregular edges around the tumor.

Mammogram with cluster microcalcifications. These clusters are usually benign, but may be cancerous.

False-negative results are also possible, particularly in women with dense breasts. In fact, a mammogram fails to detect 10 to 20 percent of cancers in these dense tissues. Ask your doctor or your mammogram technician if you have dense breast tissue. If the answer is yes, your doctor may agree to order additional tests, such as ultrasonography, MRIs, or a 3-D mammogram.

Abnormal mammogram findings that must be investigated include:

- *A white, starburst-shaped (spiculated) mass or nodule.* These are different from the clear, smooth edges of harmless cysts and benign tumors.
- *Uneven density.* Dense areas in the breast are thicker than normal and whiter than the surrounding tissue. If these densities are larger in one breast, or appear in a different part of one breast than in the other, they may be cause for concern.
- *Microcalcifications.* These calcium particles are common and usually benign, but if clustered in a certain way, they might indicate cancer.
- Any change since your previous mammogram.

Thermography

Think of thermography as a "thermal mammogram." While a mammogram uses low-dose X-ray technology, thermography produces an infrared image that shows heat and blood flow within the breasts. This test can be used to screen for breast cancer; however, the FDA is very clear in its assessment: thermography is not as sensitive as mammography and it should never be used to replace standard mammography. Mammogram is still the most reliable tool for detecting early-stage breast cancers.

Ultrasonography

We have seen that mammography is a highly useful diagnostic test but it is not foolproof. When both mammography and ultrasonography are used, a clearer picture can emerge.

Ultrasonography bounces sound waves off tissues and organs. The sound waves bounce back as patterns of echoes, which can be converted to images and projected onto a computer monitor. The procedure is painless, and you won't hear or see either the sound waves or the echoes.

To gather these images, an ultrasonography technician spreads a gel on your breast so that the sound waves can pass through more easily. Then he or she will pass a microphone-like device, called a *transducer,* over your skin. The transducer both emits the sound waves and transmits the echoes to the computer.

According to some researchers, mammography plus ultrasonography can find about 17 percent more tumors than mammography alone. Sometimes, ultrasonography can detect whether a lump in the breast is filled with fluid and most likely is a cyst, or if it is solid tissue that might or might not be cancer.

Magnetic Resonance Imaging (MRI)

Magnetic resonance imaging (MRI) uses powerful magnets and radio waves to produce computer images of body tissues. These images reveal the blood vessels in different types of tissue. Cancer spreads by forming new blood vessels, and cancer tissues contain many more blood vessels than normal tissues.

Hundreds of images are taken during an MRI, each representing a thin slice of tissue. A computer combines the images, which are read and interpreted by a radiologist.

If you are having MRI to detect breast cancer, you will probably be injected with a dye that is absorbed more quickly by cancerous tissue—where more blood vessels

---

When to Have MRI Screening for Breast Cancer

An MRI is recommended in addition to a mammogram if you:

- have a strong family history of breast or ovarian cancer
- have been determined to have an increased lifetime risk of breast cancer
- have dense breast tissue and a previous breast cancer was not detected by mammogram
- have had radiation to the chest between the ages of 10 and 30
- have a close relative who has had any of these syndromes:
  - Cowden Syndrome—a rare disorder, causing noncancerous tumors on the skin or in the lining of the mouth and nose
  - Li-Fraumeni Syndrome (LFS)—a hereditary predisposition to cancer
  - Bannayan-Riley-Ruvalcaba Syndrome (BRR)—an uncommon condition, causing noncancerous polyps of the small and large intestines

Source: American Cancer Society

---

cluster—than by normal tissue or benign tumors. The radiologist will look for concentrations of this dye that might suggest a malignancy.

MRI can be an extremely useful and accurate diagnostic tool. However, as with any test, false-positive and false-negative results are possible. For example, some nonmalignant tumors are highly vascular (have many arteries and veins) and can appear to be malignant on MRI. Likewise, slow-growing cancers with relatively few blood vessels may look like normal tissue and yield false-negative results.

MRI is painless but can be time-consuming (thirty minutes to two hours) and noisy. (The noise is the result of vibrations created when electricity creates a magnetic field inside the machine's metal coils.) You'll need to lie still most of the time as your bed moves slowly through a large cylinder. Ask your doctor how long the MRI will take and whether you can listen to music or an audiobook through the headphones provided. If you're claustrophobic, your doctor will probably prescribe medication to relax you without putting you to sleep.

Diagnosing with Biopsy

If other tests haven't ruled out cancer, you and your doctor will schedule a biopsy—an outpatient procedure in which cells, tissue sample, or an entire tumor is removed from the body for microscopic examination. Then, a *pathologist*—a doctor who diagnoses disease from tissue or blood samples—examines the sample under a microscope, and may perform other tests on it as well, to see if cancer cells are present.

It's important for the physician who performs your biopsy to remove ample tissue from the sites where cancer is suspected. A biopsy can give a precise diagnosis and is the only sure way to establish whether a lump is malignant. For a tumor to be pronounced benign, the clinical exam, the mammogram, and the biopsy must all support such a finding. For a cancer diagnosis, the biopsy alone is conclusive.

You should insist on a biopsy for any persistent or questionable lump, regardless of your family medical history or level of risk. It is your right to do so, even if others try to convince you that a clinical examination is sufficient.

Types of Biopsies

There are several types of biopsies. The one your doctor recommends may depend on the size and exact location of the lump, the number of suspicious areas in the breast, and your own preference. Asking questions ahead of time, such as the ones suggested below, may lessen any anxiety you may feel about your biopsy.

- Which type of biopsy should I have?
- Will I be awake during the biopsy?
- How much tissue will be removed?
- What tests will be performed on the tissue sample?

- What are the risks and possible side effects of my biopsy?
- When and where will I learn the results and who will report them to me?

The three major types of biopsies are fine-needle aspiration, core biopsy, and surgical biopsy. Most biopsies are performed using a local anesthetic, which numbs the area from which the sample will be taken. Occasionally, more-extensive biopsies are done with a patient under anesthesia. Note that the type of biopsy performed may vary among doctors.

Fine-Needle Aspiration

This type of biopsy, a *fine-needle aspiration (FNA),* is the least invasive type of biopsy. It is used when lumps can be easily felt and located. The FNA procedure removes a small sample of cells through a narrow, hypodermic-type needle. Your doctor will insert the biopsy needle into the lump or thickening, then will draw fluid into the syringe. A specialized pathologist, called a *cytologist,* examines cells for the presence of disease. If no cancer cells are found, your doctor may double-check the results with a more extensive biopsy, withdrawing a larger tissue sample from a lump.

Core Biopsy

The biopsy preferred by many doctors, the core biopsy takes a small, cylindrical sample of tissue from the lump rather than withdrawing only fluid. If the lump can be felt, the biopsy needle is inserted directly into it, without computer guidance. If the doctor can't feel the lump, the physician will use computer imaging or ultrasound to guide the needle. This type of procedure is referred to as *image-guided* or *stereotactic core biopsy.*

A core biopsy that is negative—one that shows no evidence of cancer—may or may not be conclusive. If there is a strong suspicion of cancer, based on an earlier imaging procedure or clinical exam, your doctor might schedule a surgical biopsy. But if your doctor believes a newly detected tumor "feels benign" to the touch and looks benign in imaging tests, then a negative core biopsy will be seen as confirming this assumption, and surgical biopsy will be unnecessary.

Another type of core biopsy is the *Mammotome*. Also called a *vacuum-assisted biopsy*, it uses a vacuum tube to gently suction breast tissue into a tube and a rotating knife removes the tissue. This procedure removes more breast tissue than in a traditional core biopsy.

Cancer brings so many issues to the table—sexual, financial, school, parenting, work. A couple who works together through these issues, which normally would be experienced over a longer period of time, will be brought closer together.

—*Holly, oncology social worker*

Surgical Biopsies

For a *surgical biopsy*, a physician removes all or part of a lump or suspicious area for examination by a pathologist. An *incisional biopsy* involves removal of a tissue sample large enough for the pathologist to make a confident diagnosis; the results of this procedure are usually conclusive. An *excisional biopsy* is, in essence, a lumpectomy—the entire lump and a small amount of the healthy tissue surrounding it are removed. Your doctor may choose excisional biopsy for small tumors that show no indications of spreading. If cancer is present, the tumor will be removed in this single procedure.

Waiting for Biopsy Results

Waiting anxiously for the results can be the worst part of a biopsy, so ask your doctor when and how you'll learn your diagnosis. At the time of your biopsy, you might want to schedule a post-biopsy appointment with your doctor to discuss the results. It's up to you. If you do have breast cancer, would you prefer to get the news in person, with a relative or a friend there to support you? The alternative might be to wait for a phone call from your doctor.

If the biopsy is positive, the combined results of all your diagnostic tests will show the characteristics of the cancer and will help your physician guide you in the best course of treatment.

Types of Breast Cancer

Breast cancer that starts in the milk ducts of the breast is called *ductal* cancer. There are two types of ductal breast cancer: ductal carcinoma *in situ* and invasive ductal carcinoma.

Ductal Carcinoma in Situ

Ductal carcinoma in situ (DCIS) is a noninvasive breast cancer. (*"In situ"* means "in the original place," meaning the cancer has not spread from the duct into surrounding tissues.) A DCIS lesion occasionally feels like a lump or a thickening of the duct, but it is more commonly detected first on a screening mammogram, where it can show up as a small cluster of calcium deposits called *microcalcifications.* However, only about 50 percent of DCIS cases develop microcalcifications that can be seen on a mammogram.

If cancer is suspected but is not visible on a mammogram, your doctor may flush out cells from the milk-duct lining and analyze them for cancer. A DCIS lesion may be discovered incidentally, when a biopsy is performed on a breast lump, or it may go undetected until it becomes invasive.

Invasive Ductal Carcinoma

If the ductal cancer has become invasive, it is referred to as *invasive ductal carcinoma.* This cancer begins growing in a milk duct and invades the fatty tissue of the breast outside of the duct. This is the most common form of breast cancer, making up about 80 percent of all cancer cases. It is usually found in a single site, not at several locations throughout the breast or in the other breast.

When I walk into a breast cancer patient's hospital room and tell her I am a ten-year survivor, I can see how good that makes her feel. I remember when I was lying in my hospital bed, I didn't think anyone survived.

—Dianna, 44

Lobular Cancer

About 10 percent of breast cancers are *lobular carcinomas.* Lobular cancer begins in the milk-producing lobules and may become invasive, spreading into surrounding breast tissue.

Lobular carcinoma is less common than ductal cancer, but has the potential to affect both breasts more than other types of breast cancer. In about 30 percent of cases, this cancer is found in both breasts; it typically feels like a thickening in the breast in the area from the nipple to the underarm. Sometimes, the skin will pucker. Lobular carcinoma does not usually show up on a mammogram. An MRI scan is recommended in cases of lobular cancer to make sure all the sites are detected.

Lobular carcinoma in situ (LCIS) refers to the presence of abnormal cells in the lobes. LCIS cells are not malignant, and the cells themselves do not develop into invasive cancer; however, these abnormal cells are signals of a risk that either lobular or ductal cancer will develop in either breast or both.

LCIS is rarely visible on a mammogram and is usually found during a biopsy on a breast lump. Treatment is bilateral mastectomy or close observation. In some cases, LCIS is treated with drugs that block the hormone estrogen, which can feed cancer cells. This form of treatment has been shown to prevent breast cancer in many high-risk women.

I highly recommend going to a breast cancer support group. You learn the tricks of the trade, hints for coping. No one really understands unless they've been through it.

—*Mary, 43*

Other Breast Cancers

There are several less common types of breast cancers, each accounting for only about 1 to 1.5 percent of all breast cancers. The *prognosis* varies among these rare cancers. Prognois refers to the likelihood of survival.

Inflammatory breast cancer is an aggressive form of the disease that is often overlooked or misdiagnosed as infection. There is usually no lump to draw attention to inflammatory breast cancer. Rather, the cancer tends to be *diffuse,* or scattered—beginning in the ducts, spreading rapidly through the lymph vessels beneath the skin, eventually blocking the flow of lymph, and sometimes spreading along the chest wall.

When symptoms appear, the breast may swell, feel warm or unusually painful, and take on a reddish tinge. The skin texture may change, developing ridges or thickening. When the skin looks pitted like the outside of an orange, the condition is known as *peau d'orange* (*"peau"* is French for skin).

Other warning signs of inflammatory breast cancer include:

- a mark like a bruise that does not go away
- nipple retraction
- bloody discharge from the nipple
- itching that isn't relieved by creams or ointments
- swelling in lymph nodes under the arm or above the collarbone

Warmth or pain in the breast, redness, and swelling are symptoms of breast infection, or *mastitis,* for which antibiotics are typically prescribed. When antibiotics don't clear up the problem, the next step is usually a biopsy.

Inflammatory breast cancer is a highly aggressive and dangerous form of the disease. It requires aggressive and immediate treatment, often in the form of chemotherapy followed by surgery, radiation therapy, additional chemotherapy, and hormonal therapy. If you have any inflammatory breast cancer symptoms, see your doctor immediately and insist on a biopsy without delay.

Tumor Characteristics

Learning the characteristics of a tumor helps oncologists determine the stage of a cancer and it also helps them determine the best course of treatment. Some details about a woman's breast cancer will be known after a biopsy; however, the fuller understanding of the cancer's characteristics will be known after the tumor is surgically removed and studied in a lab.

Size of a Tumor

Small tumors measure up to two centimeters (less than an inch) in diameter. Medium-size tumors are between two and five centimeters (up to two inches), and large tumors are more than five centimeters (two inches).

Cancer Cells in Blood Vessels or Lymph Vessels

Because blood and lymph fluid circulate throughout the body, they can carry cancer cells almost anywhere. Thus, cancer cells in the blood vessels or lymph vessels signify a greater likelihood of metastasis (spreading) to other parts of the body.

Appearance of the Cancer Cells

As normal cells mature, they take on distinctive, specialized shapes, depending on their function. Under a

---

Gene Mutations

Genes are short segments of DNA—the body's blueprint for cell development and function. Mutations in certain cells can occur at some point in a person's life. The mutations may be the result of heredity or environmental factors; or an error may occur as cells are dividing. If a healthy cell does not repair the mutation, it can increast the risk for cancer.

BRCA1: this gene normally repairs cells. However, if the gene becomes damaged *(mutated)*, it increases the risk of several cancers: breast, ovarian, pancreatic, cervical, uterine, and colon. However, the main increased risk is for breast and ovarian cancer. A parent can pass a mutated gene on to a child.

BRCA2: this gene performs the same tasks as the BRCA1 gene, but if it becomes damaged, it increases the risk for breast cancer, ovarian cancer, pancreatic cancer, and melanoma. This mutation can be hereditary.

PALB2: a gene that works with BRCA2 proteins to repair cells and stop tumor growth. However, a mutated PALB2 gene increases the risk of breast cancer. PALB2 stands for partner and localizer for the BRCA2 gene. Some of the other more common gene mutations that increase the risk of breast cancer include: RAD51C, CHEK2, ATM, and PTEN.

---

microscope, mature breast cells look very different from, say, mature skin cells or liver cells.

Well-differentiated breast cancer cells are typical of slow-growing cancers. They look much like normal, mature breast cells, with clearly defined boundaries. Poorly differentiated breast cancer cells are very different in appearance—they have "uneven," indistinct boundaries. These cells are found in aggressive tumors.

Hormone and Cellular Receptor Status

Hormone receptor status refers to whether breast cancer cells have receptors for the hormones estrogen and progesterone. *Hormone receptors* are proteins found in and on breast cells that pick up hormone signals telling the cells to grow. In diagnosing breast cancer, doctors look for receptors for the hormones *estrogen* and *progesterone.* These hormones circulate throughout a woman's body

Cellular Receptors

Some breast cancer cells have receptors on the outside of their cells to which the female hormones estrogen and progesterone can attach. These hormones can fuel breast cancer growth by triggering cellular mutations.

Estrogen receptor: these receptors use the hormone estrogen to grow. Cancer with these receptors is called estrogen positive (ER+).

Progesterone receptor: these receptors use the hormone progesterone to grow. Cancer with these receptors is referred to as progesterone positive (PR+).

Hormone receptor negative: these cancer cells do not have receptors that attract the hormones estrogen or progesterone. They are referred to as hormone receptor negative (HR-).

HER2 status: HER2 is a gene that controls normal breast cell growth. However, if the gene becomes damaged, it can make too much of the HER2 protein, which can promote cancer growth. Cancers that have high levels of HER2 receptors on the cells are referred to as HER2 positive (HER2+).

Triple negative: this form of breast cancer lacks all three types of cell receptors, estrogen, progesterone, or HER2.

but interact only with cells that have the receptors to which the hormones can attach themselves.

Testing cancer cells for estrogen and progesterone receptors can help doctors understand how aggressive a cancer might be and what kinds of treatment would be most effective. If your breast cancer has a significant number of receptors for estrogen, it means the cancer may receive signals from estrogen that promote cancer growth. This type of cancer is called *estrogen receptor positive (ER+).* Similarly, if the cancer cells have a significant number of receptors for progesterone, it means the cancer is receiving signals from progesterone to continue growing. This is called *progesterone receptor positive (PR+).* If a cancer has few or no such hormone receptors, it is called *hormone-receptor negative.*

Another factor in assessing breast cancer cellular receptors is the HER2 gene. This gene is a factor in 20 to 30 percent of breast cancers; it "tells" cells to grow and divide, but sometimes a gene defect occurs, which creates too many HER2 proteins and receptors for HER2 on the cell. This results in cells growing too quickly, leading to a fast-growing tumor in the breast tissue. Breast tumors that are HER2+ *(positive)* have excess HER2 and are more aggressive than tumors that are HER2- *(negative).*

If breast cancer is positive for estrogen, progesterone, or HER2, treatment may include hormone- or HER2-blocking drugs. As the name of these drugs suggests, these treatments block the hormones or HER2 from feeding the cancer cells.

Some breast cancers lack any receptors for estrogen, progesterone, or HER2. This type of cancer is known as *triple negative* breast cancer, and it can grow aggressively. Because it has no hormone receptors, it does not respond to hormone-blocking therapies; however, chemotherapies can be effective in treatment.

Testing Tumor Tissue

In addition to testing for hormone status and cellular receptor status, your oncologist will likely order other tests on tumor tissue. Like other testing, these tests help determine how aggressive a cancer is and which course of treatment will be most effective.

For example, a test may be performed on tumor tissue to check for a mutation of the *p53 gene.* This gene monitors cell growth to limit how quickly cells divide into new cells. When this gene is damaged, cells can grow out of control, and a tumor can form.

Tumor tissue may also be tested for the *Ki-67 protein.* The test helps determine whether a cancer is growing aggressively. If many cells are expressing the protein, a tumor is growing quickly. If very few cells express this protein, a cancer is growing slowly.

The Ki-67 test is commonly performed prior to chemotherapy or radiation and then again after such treatments to determine whether the treatment is effective or needs to be changed.

Stages of Breast Cancer

After your doctor knows exactly where the cancer is, additional tests will determine its stage—in other words, whether it has been caught early, late, or somewhere in between. Three characteristics determine the stage of a cancer: its size, its aggressiveness, and its location in sites other than the original tumor. The likelihood of survival (the patient's *prognosis*) can depend on the stage at which the cancer is diagnosed.

Doctors use a variety of tests for cancer staging—a blood test for liver metastases, a chest X-ray for metastases to the lung, or a PET or CT scan to gather additional information about the disease at the cellular level. Another test, a *sentinel node biopsy,* gives doctors the ability to detect even small numbers of cancer cells. This test involves sampling an underarm node called the *sentinel node,* which is usually the first node to receive lymph drainage from the breast tumor. Therefore, it is the first node in which spreading cancer cells are likely to appear. This test makes it possible to stage breast cancer more accurately. As a result, sentinel node biopsy has become the standard staging procedure for breast cancer, though it is by no means the only one. (*See* chapter 4 for further discussion of sentinel node biopsy.)

Also, at the time of cancer surgery, the doctor may withdraw bone-marrow cells to be examined for evidence of *micrometastases,* free-floating cancer cells that have not yet formed a mass.

After all the information about your cancer is collected, it will be staged as one of these levels: 0, I, II, III, or IV. The staging guidelines are complex: your oncologist will explain the stage of your cancer to you.

Testing for Risk of Recurrence

Whether or not a cancer spreads depends partially on the behavior of genes within the tumor. Thanks to technology, newer tests are now available to examine the genes of breast cancer tissue. These tests serve as indicators of whether a woman's risk of recurrence is low or high. Accordingly, the test results help doctors and patients choose the best line of postsurgical treatment. For example, if the risk is low, doctors may recommend hormone therapy. If the risk is high, doctors may recommend a more aggressive treatment that includes chemotherapy.

One such test, *MammaPrint,* is used to evaluate tumor tissue. This genetic test assesses seventy-one genes and determines the likelihood of cancer recurring within five to ten years of the initial diagnosis. MammaPrint can be used to test women under age sixty who have stage I or stage II breast cancer with negative nodes and tumors no larger than five centimeters (two inches).

Another test, *Oncotype DX,* provides information for pre- and postmenopausal women with early-stage (stage I or II ER+) breast cancer. The test assesses twenty-one genes and indicates whether a woman is at low or high risk for recurrence.

3

COPING EMOTIONALLY

If you're like most women, when you heard the words "breast cancer," you may have feared the worst. Perhaps you have memories from years ago about family members or friends who died from the disease. But, thanks to medical advances, this much-feared disease is no longer equated with imminent death. Although it is a life-threatening disease, breast cancer has become a treatable cancer, and many women who develop it are living long lives.

Meanwhile, it's normal to feel a barrage of emotions upon receiving a diagnosis. Shock, fear for yourself, fear for your family, denial, and panic are all common reactions. Suddenly, you have to gather and absorb a great deal of information you never dreamed you'd need.

Sometimes you may feel overwhelmed. But you will learn to manage these new demands and to honor your feelings. You will develop strategies for coping. Soon, your own, unique style of coping will become part of the wisdom breast cancer patients are eager to share; sooner than you think, you may be helping others down the road you're traveling today.

Find Support

Studies indicate that the diagnostic phase is an extremely stressful time for women with breast cancer. Experts say talking with others about an illness helps to relieve some of the stress. Some women turn to their significant others, relatives, or close friends. There are also a number of other ways you can find support that will help you through this worrisome time in your life.

Meet with Your Doctor

Your primary care doctor—the one you see for routine health care—may be an excellent initial source of information. Make an appointment to see him or her as soon as possible after your diagnosis. Here are some tips to prepare for your first appointment.

- Write down all your questions. Give a copy to the doctor and keep one for yourself. That way, you won't be tempted to skip some of the questions if you feel you're taking up too much of the doctor's time.
- Do some research on your own before your appointment if it eases your mind. The more you know beforehand, the more new information you can absorb during your conversation.
- Don't expect to be on top of things right away. There's a lot to learn.
- Invite your mate or a close friend to go with you. He or she can take notes and help you remember the discussion in detail.

Conduct Your Own Research

Not all your questions about breast cancer will be answered during the first meeting with your doctor. New questions will come up. Jot them down as they occur to you. Books, articles, and websites offer vast amounts of information, from the general to the specific.

Familiarize yourself with the library, local bookstores, and the Internet. You'll find dozens of books on breast cancer, ranging from the very technical and scientific to simple presentations of pertinent facts. Decide how much

---

Questions to Ask Your Physician

- What kind of breast cancer do I have?
- Will I lose my breast?
- What are my chances for long-term survival?
- Are further tests needed to find out whether the cancer has spread?
- How will I know which course of treatment is best for me?
- When will I begin treatment?
- How long will it take to recover from surgery and other treatments?
- Can you suggest support groups or services that might help me and my family?

---

you want to know and then look for publications that will meet your needs.

If you have access to the Internet, you'll find thousands of sites that publish material online, offer books and pamphlets for sale, or both. You'll also find breast cancer organizations, chat rooms, support groups, and inspiring stories of other women who have, or have had, breast cancer. These can be enormously comforting and helpful to you at every phase of dealing with the disease. If you don't have a computer or you're unfamiliar with the Internet, most libraries have public computers and staff who can show you how to use them.

Be careful about the websites you visit. Not all are accurate and up to date. Make sure the site sponsor is reputable. If you come across confusing or conflicting information, ask your doctor about it.

Meet with a Survivor

Breast cancer survivors say that one of the most important things you can do for yourself is meet face-to-face with at least one woman who has been successfully treated for breast cancer. Find someone who has a positive attitude and who is a good listener. You might already know someone who fits that description, or your doctor can refer you to patients he or she has treated who would be willing to talk with you. Online conversations are all well and good, but your computer can't give you a hug, hand you a tissue, or hold your hand.

I feel like I've been able to help others through my own breast cancer. All of my coworkers had mammograms right after I was diagnosed. One of them found she had a malignancy in the very early stages.

—Joan, 47

Minimize Outside Obligations

Life goes on, even if you aren't able to in your usual fashion. Some women continue with all their activities during breast cancer treatment; others decide to scale back a little, or a lot. You may need to rethink your professional and community responsibilities. If you serve on committees or boards, or lead a scout troop, or volunteer at a homeless shelter, let people know if you need to be out of commission for a while and that someone else will have to fill in for you.

At your job, try to anticipate problems and prepare for them. Work with your employer to find a temporary replacement for the times you can't be there. Check to see how much sick leave you can take, what your employer's extended-leave policy is, and whether you have long-term care insurance. You might not need a long absence from work, but it's good to know how to arrange one if necessary.

If your employer is uncooperative, remember that state laws and the federal *Americans with Disabilities Act* and *Family Medical Leave Act* exist to protect your job, your benefits, your seniority, and your status, and require your employer to provide "reasonable accommodation" to you during your treatment and recovery. These laws apply to most public agencies and all but the smallest private employers. (Some federal employees are covered by a different law.)

For details on your legal rights under state and federal law and to receive an informative booklet, contact the American Cancer Society (*See* the Resources section at the back of this book).

Be Involved in Your Treatment

The level of your involvement in your treatment really is up to you. The questions that are most important to you, and your urgency in getting them answered, will serve as a guide. Bit by bit, you'll discover whether you want detailed information about every procedure, medication, and treatment option, or whether you're content to know only enough to be an informed patient.

Take your time deciding how involved you want to be—then feel free to change your mind. Maybe at first you'll want to be a walking breast cancer encyclopedia, but later, after getting to know and trust your cancer specialist, decide you are satisfied with just a grasp of the general principles.

Seek Emotional and Psychological Support

Think about coping strategies that have helped you keep your balance in the past. You can rely on this inner strength now. But if your coping skills aren't up to the task, your doctor, your research, and your support system can help.

It's natural to experience powerful and sometimes conflicting emotions after a diagnosis of breast cancer. Acknowledge your feelings and give them room. Confide in people who will listen and understand—even when your feelings are difficult to describe—and avoid well-meaning friends who try to talk you out of feeling the way you do.

Do not deny your emotions, no matter how inappropriate they might seem at first. Who knows?

Tuning in to your most turbulent emotions, and surrendering to quietly pensive feelings as well, might surprise you with moments of great joy, even in the midst of sorrow and anger. Life warrants all these feelings, and more, and a crisis such as breast cancer can bring all of life into sharp focus.

Your goal of feeling strong and at peace is not well served if you explode in anger over small things, take your fears out on others, or pretend to be on top of things when you're not. As with most situations, a balanced and honest approach is the most effective.

I had friends who had breast cancer and they really got me through the tough times. I would lay out all my fears and one of them would always have something funny to say about it. We would just howl. It's hard to be afraid of something when you can laugh at it.

—Ann, 53

Find creative ways to uncover and release your emotions. Writing, making music, dancing, drawing, painting, doing home improvement projects, gardening, and even cooking can be excellent ways to express your feelings and create something worthwhile in the process. Conversation—intimate, confidential talk with your spouse, partner, or a friend—can be healing and strengthening if that person is supportive.

If your emotions seem out of control, however, and nothing has helped, consider getting professional counseling. Ask your doctor to refer you to someone who specializes in working with cancer patients, especially those with breast cancer.

Strong emotion is not inappropriate. Tears and anger are normal and even healthy ways to keep from bottling up your feelings. Allow yourself to cry and grieve. Give yourself permission to be angry. As long as your anger isn't unleashed on them, the people who care about you should accept it and not scold you for "giving in to it." The most uncomfortable feelings of sadness and anger will be resolved sooner if you plod on through them rather than try to sneak around them.

Choose the appropriate time and place to punch pillows or shout yourself hoarse. Let your anger become the energy that pushes you to learn, take charge, take care of yourself, hang on to humor, and hope. But if, instead of releasing your anger, you end up feeling angrier than ever, consider it a sign that you could benefit from counseling or a therapeutic support group.

You might think the feelings that surge inside you have never been experienced by anyone else. The truth is, you're not alone. Others have felt, or are feeling right now, the very same emotions.

Join a Support Group

Other breast cancer patients can offer you validation and hope. They can understand your feelings and experiences. In fact, your support group might become vitally important, if only to relieve your feelings of isolation. Knowing you are not alone can give you great comfort.

Breast cancer support groups are made up of women of all ages and from all walks of life. Most large hospitals offer support groups specifically for women with breast cancer. Those who take advantage of these groups report that the meetings and the new relationships give them strength. Hearing others express fears, celebrate triumphs (large or small), and share valuable information can be healing and calming. Sadly, the women who could profit most from a support group—those who are the most depressed, anxious, and fearful—often don't join one.

The National Cancer Institute's Cancer Information Service, the American Cancer Society, and your hospital or breast cancer clinic can help you find appropriate support groups that meet face-to-face or online. The National Coalition for Cancer Survivorship helps cancer

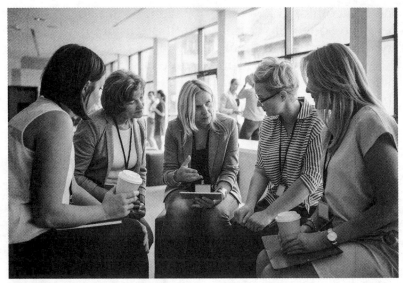

Other breast cancer patients understand your experience. Support groups offer an environment for emotional healing.

survivors and their families start local support groups or contact existing ones. For information about contacting these organizations, *see* the Resources section at the back of this book.

Explore Your Spirituality

Some women already have strong religious faith or spirituality when they learn that they have breast cancer, or they soon find themselves drawn toward greater spirituality. Others rely on their own grit and self-reliance to see them through.

If you are spiritually inclined, your experience with breast cancer could deepen your faith. Talking with a minister, rabbi, priest, or other spiritual adviser about your illness may offer comfort. It can also become an opportunity to learn more about what you believe, what you fear, and what your particular faith teaches about God, mortality, the self, and the most meaningful way to live.

Most of these questions concern everyone, whether or not they profess religious faith, so they are worth your contemplation. If you are not religious, talking with those who are can be enlightening. You can also find wisdom in the works of nonreligious thinkers and in poetry, art, literature, and nature. Finding ways to look beyond the boundaries of your own life—perhaps seeing order and purpose there—can bring you peace and comfort. It is the kind of comfort that comes from feeling yourself as a small—but not smaller than others—part of an immense and very grand universe.

When my mom first told me about her cancer, I was worried. Who would take care of me? What if she dies? She was totally honest with me. That was reassuring.

—*Gail, 13*

Practice Meditation, Good Nutrition, and Exercise

One way to quiet your mind and relieve your anxiety is to meditate. Spending just ten to twenty minutes, twice a day, in a deeply relaxed and focused state not only confers a sense of tranquility but also helps the body fight the damaging effects of stress.

Some women meditate by silently repeating the word "peace" while calmly releasing any distractions that arise in their mind. Others use a form of meditation called *visualization* or *guided imagery*. In a state of deep relaxation, they picture the body healing itself. They intently visualize their cancer shrinking, their immune cells fighting like microscopic armies against cancer cells, their energy returning, their color radiant, their life in balance.

If meditation appeals to you, learn more about it through your research on the Internet or in publications. Consider taking a class in meditation or yoga. Some styles of yoga use stretches, movement, and body postures to promote a meditative state. Others focus more on yoga as exercise. Either style can calm and energize you. In fact, any activity that lifts your spirits and supports your overall health will improve both your mental and physical well-being.

Eating healthfully is another way to fight your cancer. A nutritious low-fat diet has been shown to decrease the risk of getting cancer. Raw foods believed to inhibit cancer growth include broccoli, cabbage, brussels sprouts, cauliflower, mustard greens, turnip greens, kale, and radishes. Animal studies have demonstrated that dietary fiber can reduce the risk of breast cancer, perhaps by preventing estrogen from stimulating the growth of breast malignancies.

More than a hundred studies have found significant decreases in cancer rates among people whose diets are high in fruits and vegetables; these foods contain vitamins A, C, and E; the minerals magnesium, zinc, phosphorous, and folic acid; and beta-carotene. Good sources of beta carotene come from apricots, beet greens, black-eyed peas, cantaloupe, carrots, sweet potatoes, pumpkin, and spinach.

Studies have not confirmed the benefits of taking vitamins, but recent research has shown that vitamin D may provide protection from diseases such as cancer, osteoporosis, hypertension, and some autoimmune diseases. Ask your doctor about the dosage that is right for you.

Women with breast cancer who exercise have improved outcomes compared to those who do not. Further, women with breast cancer who exercised during treatment reported that they had more energy and did not gain as much weight as those who didn't exercise. (Some women lose weight during treatment; others gain weight. *See* more on weight changes in chapter 7.) Exercise such as walking, swimming, dance, or other programs can offer a physical and emotional boost.

Put Your Own Needs First

This really isn't as selfish as it sounds. In the long run, everybody will be better off because you took care of yourself when you needed to. Even so, it's difficult for many women to hand off their responsibilities. We are society's caretakers, its wives and mothers, and usually its nurses, secretaries, child-care workers, and schoolteachers. We tend to put our loved ones' needs before our own. A breast cancer diagnosis can require a sudden reversal of lifelong habits, which at first will likely be yet another source of stress.

Let people close to you be helpful. Explain to your family and friends that you must put all your energy into your treatment—not only your surgery and therapies, but also learning, resting, and staying focused, which will help you keep your spirits up.

Addressing the Needs of Others

Throughout your treatment, you'll naturally be concerned about the people close to you. Putting yourself first doesn't mean ignoring your friends and family, especially your children. Though most of your active tending to others' needs might need to wait until your treatments have ended, there are ways to help without immersing yourself in their care.

As much as you want to spare your family and friends any pain, worry, or inconvenience, in one way or another your breast cancer will affect everyone around you. Your husband or life partner, especially, is likely to experience intense emotions. Your children's reactions will depend on their age, personality, gender, and stage of emotional development. Your friends, especially women close to you in age, will not only be concerned about you but might also be somewhat anxious, knowing that they, too, could develop breast cancer.

Some people will know instinctively how to comfort you and offer help. Most will not, at least at first. Some never will be able to. There is no "right way" for someone to react to your illness. Try not to judge or be hurt when friends or relatives are awkward around you or even avoid you. It doesn't mean they don't care. It's just that everyone copes differently and expresses emotions in different ways.

The following sections describe what the people in your life might be going through and how you can acknowledge their struggles without letting them wear you down.

After working with breast cancer patients for fourteen years, I've found that patients connecting with other patients is the key to coping. Patients sharing their journeys is the best medicine.

—*Ann, oncology social worker*

Spouses and Partners

If your spouse or partner is the strong, silent type, he or she may hesitate to discuss their feelings for fear of burdening you. They might go into denial about your disease, or might overcompensate by being excessively cheerful. The more you share your feelings and needs with your partner, the better they may be able to face their own. You might need to give your partner explicit permission to open up emotionally. But perhaps they can't do that, or provide the support you need, no matter how much they love you. Sometimes people just get mired in feelings of fear, sadness, anger, or helplessness in the face of their partner's disease.

Letting your partner know that you don't blame them—and that you are not without support from friends, clergy, a counselor, or a support group—could help them deal with their own emotions. Eventually, they might learn how to help you by helping themself. Or they might not, in which case you can choose to accept them the way they are. The alternative—a constant, smoldering resentment—will be at least as harmful to you as to your partner.

Remind relatives and friends that they can make a world of difference by offering a kind word, babysitting, or otherwise sharing responsibility with your partner. Looking back, many partners say they would simply like to have been asked, "How are you doing?"

If your partner asks, "What can I do to help you?" take him or her up on the offer and suggest something constructive—some activity that will reduce your anxiety.

Children

Children of every age, newborn to adult, are profoundly affected by a mother's breast cancer. Even infants are attuned to their parents' emotions and unsettled by the secrecy surrounding illness. The best thing you can do is accept their natural reactions to your cancer. Answer their questions with as much or as little information as they can absorb at their age and level of development. It might help them to confide in a trusted adult who isn't caught up in the crisis—a school counselor, teacher, neighbor, pastor, or friend.

Babies and Toddlers

The youngest children often respond to parents' stress by crying more, needing more attention, eating less, and sleeping poorly. Hold and comfort them as often as possible. Try to keep them on a consistent schedule. If they have begun to talk, give them very simple information ("Mommy's sick") and prepare them for changes in the household routine ("She might have to go away for a few days to get better").

Children Ages Three to Six

At these ages, children do not yet have reasoning skills and can see things only from their own point of view. They might think they caused the cancer or they might worry about getting sick themselves. Since young children tend to fear separation, prepare them for your absences. When neither parent can be with them, they should be cared for (preferably at home, where they feel safe) by someone they know well and trust.

Because they don't understand their emotions, they might act out—throwing tantrums, hitting, pushing, crying. Try to maintain their daily routine. Calmly, in simple terms, explain any changes from that routine. Comfort them, reassure them that they are not at fault, and acknowledge that they might feel sad or scared.

Children Ages Seven to Eleven

By these ages, children are beginning to think logically. Capable of reasoning, they are also capable of understanding (and fearing) the finality of death. They'll be most anxious about the immediate future, however. They might worry about the tangible effects of your cancer, such as the cost of medical care or the welfare of younger siblings. Acknowledge their fears and other feelings, and assure them that adults have these matters well in hand.

Always be truthful, without giving them more information than they can grasp. If you can't promise you'll recover, give them realistic reasons for hope, such as treatment advances, new discoveries through research, and inspirational stories about women who have beaten the odds.

Adolescent Children

From age twelve through their teenage years, children experience rapid physical, psychological, and emotional changes that make them extremely vulnerable. Because they are trying hard to establish their independence, develop their own identity, and separate from parents and childhood, they typically deny their vulnerability. Teenagers cling to self-absorption—the way a bud seems to hold itself tightly before it flowers—and think that bad things happen to other people, not to them.

Their mother's illness can undermine this certainty and draw them back into childhood and dependency. Be sensitive to this. Ask them to help out in tangible ways, recognizing that they are approaching adulthood but still have one foot in childhood. Talk about your own feelings in ways they can understand and deal with. This might prompt them to do likewise. But don't push. Sometimes, just being together is more reassuring than serious talk.

Adult Children

Your grown children will want to know how they can help, whether they live nearby or on another continent. No matter what their ages, a mother's serious illness can awaken long-forgotten feelings of dependence and deep anxiety, which may in turn trigger the need to control.

A son, for example, who typically uses his competence to deal with uncertainty, might want to take charge of your care. Welcome his concern, share information with him, but firmly assure him that you are capable of making all the necessary decisions.

Daughters are likely to worry about their own susceptibility to breast cancer, as well they should. Emphasize the importance of monthly breast self-examination and annual checkups. Express the hope that your breast cancer diagnosis will actually reduce their own risk by making them more conscientious about preventive care.

Other Family Members, Friends, and Acquaintances

Members of your extended family will naturally feel the impact of your cancer in different ways. Your parents may fear for you as they did when you were a child, and you might find your traditional roles turned upside-down as they look to you for comfort and reassurance.

Your siblings, besides being worried, will also feel a bit fragile themselves. If you are the first person of your generation to have cancer, they'll be awakened to their own vulnerability. If your cancer is hereditary, your sisters will have to confront their own breast cancer risk and that of their daughters. These concerns may seem selfish, but they also are quite realistic and they certainly don't diminish your siblings' love for you or their compassion for your struggle.

Family and friends will deal with your illness in ways that reflect their personalities, character, emotional makeup, and just plain busy-ness. Don't be offended by those who don't call or visit as often as others or who are less forthcoming with food, favors, and willingness to sit and talk with you. Some people have no idea what to do or say. Let them know that you understand, that it helps just to know they care, and that you're still interested in their day-to-day goings-on. Your reassurance might free them to show their concern more openly.

Sexuality and Intimacy

There's no medical reason to delay having sex after breast surgery unless your doctor advises otherwise. But you might not be particularly interested in sex right away, for a variety of reasons. For one thing, you've just had surgery and you'll be gathering your strength for a while. On top of that, your nonsurgical therapy—radiation, chemotherapy, hormonal therapy, or another treatment—can temporarily dampen your desire, tire you, or cause other symptoms (such as vaginal dryness) that are likely to bump sexual activity off the top of your priority list.

After a mastectomy, with or without breast reconstruction, you have an entirely new body image to adjust to, and it will take some time for you to feel sexy and appealing. At the same time, you may fear your partner's reaction to your altered anatomy or that your partner might be reluctant to approach you for fear of causing you physical pain. If you're not communicating, it's easy to draw the wrong conclusions, each of you perhaps thinking the other is indifferent.

My doctor found my breast cancer during a routine mammogram shortly after I turned 40. I immediately started to cry and thought I was going to die, but I didn't.

—*Alice, 46*

For some couples, unacknowledged barriers to intimacy are a serious threat to the relationship. A discussion with your doctor might be helpful for the two of you. The doctor can explain to what extent your problem might be physiological, caused by treatment-induced hormonal changes, and to what extent it is emotional. He or she can reassure your partner that having sex won't cause you physical injury. And your doctor or a counselor can open the lines of communication between the two of you. Clearly, communication is crucial here. If the two of you don't share your fears openly, there's a lot of room for misunderstanding. Keeping quiet about anxieties will only push them deeper.

Assure your partner that you find him desirable. Tell him about your insecurities, and encourage him to share his feelings as well. Most husbands prove to be loving, supportive, and accepting of their wives' changed bodies and their topsy-turvy feelings.

Until you are energetic and confident enough to have intercourse, you can maintain closeness by cuddling, holding, caressing, and confiding in one another. Without question, do not have sex until you're ready. Experts are unanimous on this point: Feeling obligated to have intercourse when you'd rather be doing almost anything else can be an ever-present source of stress and guilt feelings, which aren't beneficial at any time but can be especially harmful to you now. Allow time for your body and spirit to heal, and look forward to a lifetime of growing, changing, and intimacy with the one you love.

Challenges after Treatment

Even cancer patients with very promising prognoses may have a need for treatment for future medical, psychological, and other issues. For example, a disease or therapy may cause damage to the heart or other organs; or, a cancer might recur years later.

The physical aftereffects, however, aren't the only concern. Approximately 70 percent of individuals undergoing cancer treatment become depressed or anxious at some point during their diagnostic and treatment periods. They also often experience fear that a cancer will return despite intensive treatment. Even reaching a milestone in recovery can trigger doubts and skepticism about the ability to stay healthy. Any physical change or symptom, for example, may raise fears that the cancer is back.

Further, survivors may experience grief over the perceived loss of their health, physical independence, self-esteem, and other aspects of their life. They also may need help in adjusting to possible changes in their relationships with family members, friends, and even coworkers. Since cancer can be an isolating experience, patients often need help in approaching others who avoid them or don't want to talk about their disease. They also may experience a renewed sense of spirituality or religious conviction or have a new sense of what is important in their life.

Cancer Survivorship Programs

A growing number of Americans are disease-free after cancer treatment. National Cancer Institute (NCI) statistics suggest more than 15.5 million Americans are living with a history of cancer. Other NCI estimates project the number of people surviving beyond their diagnosis will reach 19 million by 2024. As more people survive cancer, survivorship programs have been developed to help individuals cope with the physical, psychological, emotional, social, and even spiritual issues that often surface even after successful treatment. These programs provide expertise, education, and other resources to help people move from cancer patient to cancer survivor.

Access to Support

A team of medical professionals and survivorship specialists help individuals identify their specific challenges and then address them with the necessary tools. That includes therapy for emotional concerns, support groups, classes, family member counseling, and access to community services and professionals.

Even though a survivorship treatment plan is unique to an individual, it will likely include:

- *Regular physical examinations.* Patients not only learn to manage possible long-term effects of their disease, but also focus on normal health maintenance in supporting their results. As part of reviewing a patient's overall health, the medical team emphasizes monitoring and screening for both new and recurring cancers.

- *Management of treatment-related side effects.* Even with successful therapy, cancer survivors may experience some residual effects of treatment that may influence their daily activities. A survivorship program gives patients tools for addressing those and other health problems. Since cancer can also affect preexisting and chronic conditions, working with specialists after treatment can be an important step in addressing any remaining health challenges related to those problems.

- *Lifestyle coaching.* Cancer survivorship programs emphasize changes that boost a person's overall well-being while reducing future cancer risks. By focusing on proper nutrition, exercise, and lifestyle choices, for instance, participants gain new tools for maximizing their health as well as continuing their success with treatment. Exercise physiologists and nutritionists are likely participants.

- *Referrals.* Although a patient's primary physicians are still central to care, survivorship programs also offer expert opinions and links to medical specialists with experience working specifically with similar patients in recovery. They can help with fertility, sexual health, and issues related to specific organs and systems in the body that might have been affected by the cancer or treatment. Survivorship programs also can be helpful sources for employment, insurance, and other financial information.

Oncology groups as well as cancer centers often provide cancer survivorship programs for their patients. The National Coalition for Cancer Survivorship offers further information (*see* the Resources section at the back of this book). By providing a continuum of care, a multidisciplinary team can help patients improve quality of life beyond their cancer treatment.

4

SURGERY FOR BREAST CANCER

Virtually every woman diagnosed with breast cancer undergoes surgery, which may or may not be followed by radiation and other therapies. Today, women with breast cancer can choose from a variety of surgical options that were not available to their mothers. And, there's good news. Early detection and modern surgical techniques have increased survival rates and helped many women avoid losing one or both breasts.

Choosing a Breast Surgeon

After a breast cancer diagnosis, your doctor will likely refer you to a breast surgeon. If you like and trust the breast surgeon to whom your doctor has referred you, great! If not, perhaps you'll want to find the surgeon who is right for you. How do you go about this?

- Ask your physician for another referral.
- Get the names of breast cancer surgeons in your area from several credible sources: friends, coworkers, physicians, nurses, and other health professionals. Find out which of these surgeons are on the staffs of highly rated hospitals. Develop a working list, then look at the doctors' credentials on their websites. Interview as many as it takes to find one whom you trust and feel comfortable with.

- Get in touch with an organization such as the National Cancer Institute (NCI), the American Cancer Society, or the American Society of Breast Surgeons. Contact information for these and other organizations appears in the Resources section at the back of this book.
- Find breast cancer hotlines or women's health groups in your area that can point you toward breast cancer specialists and other resources.

First Meeting with a Breast Surgeon

Many women feel overwhelmed by unfamiliar medical terms and decisions to make at a time when they are already emotionally overwrought. For this reason, it's a good idea to take your partner or a close friend with you when you first meet with your surgeon. Have your companion take notes so that you need not remember all the new information laid out before you. Later, you and your companion can review the conversation with the surgeon.

If a surgeon believes you will need additional treatment after your surgery, he or she can refer you to other specialists, such as a radiation oncologist, who oversees radiation therapy, or a medical oncologist, who oversees chemotherapy. As before, you don't have to accept a surgeon's recommendations and may wish to evaluate each doctor on your own. In general, a specialist who is ethical, experienced, and attuned to your needs is one who:

- shows genuine concern for you and is not overly clinical or detached
- is a good teacher, explaining things thoroughly but clearly, in language you can readily understand
- takes a detailed history and performs a complete physical exam
- asks how you're feeling emotionally

- has considerable experience with cases like yours
- is up to date on the newest treatments and research
- welcomes the involvement of family members or a close friend
- supports the use of all necessary pain management
- patiently answers all your questions and does not regard any of them as unimportant
- notices when you're confused or anxious and tactfully draws you out
- encourages you to get a second opinion on any treatment decision

Questions for Your Surgeon

You will no doubt have questions about your surgery. When it comes to your breast cancer and its treatments, there's no such thing as an inappropriate question. Ask your surgeon about anything that concerns you, though it might not be possible to answer some of your questions until after surgery. Here are some sample questions to help you start your own list:

- Will I need radiation therapy, chemotherapy, hormonal therapy, or targeted therapy following my surgery?
- What side effects can I expect from surgery?
- Will my surgery be done on an outpatient basis, or will I be hospitalized? If so, for how long?
- When should I have breast reconstruction—at the time of surgery or later?
- Will I have drainage tubes?
- When will I be able to go back to work?
- Will my physical activities be restricted? For how long?
- Will I need physical therapy?

Discuss Surgical Incisions and Scars

Before your breast surgery, talk with your surgeon about the incision or incisions that will be used. If you are having a partial mastectomy, you will want to know how much scarring to expect and how the surgeon will keep scarring to a minimum. Ask whether the shape and direction of the incision can affect your remaining breast tissue—Will it pucker? Will your scar pull the nipple out of its normal position or show above a bathing suit? After surgery, will you have any concave areas in your breast?

If your entire breast will be removed and you want to have reconstruction, ask how much of your skin and nipple can be spared for the reconstruction process and how the incision will be positioned to allow for the best cosmetic outcome.

Techniques for hiding or minimizing scars are continually improving. For example, because the nipple position and weight distribution are completely different in upright positions, surgeons now decide on placement of incisions based on the appearance of a woman's breasts when she is standing, sitting, and walking, rather than during an examination, when she is lying down.

Types of Breast Surgery

The type of breast surgery your surgeon recommends depends on several factors, including the type, stage, and location of the cancer. Other factors include your feelings about breast preservation or reconstruction, your prognosis, genetic risks, and your general health.

Overall, complications with breast cancer surgeries are rare. Hospital stays depend on the surgery being performed and whether any reconstruction will be done. Lumpectomies are typically performed on an outpatient basis. For other procedures, most stays are overnight; if complex reconstruction surgery is performed the stay may be longer—two to six days.

Partial Mastectomy

When a portion of the breast is removed during surgery, the procedure is called a *partial mastectomy*. There are two major types of partial mastectomy—lumpectomy and quadrantectomy. The difference between them is the amount of the breast that is removed. Partial mastectomies are usually outpatient procedures, even with lymph node removal.

Lumpectomy. For a *lumpectomy* procedure, a surgeon removes the tumor and some of the surrounding healthy tissue. The whole breast is not removed.

The lumpectomy procedure is possible when a tumor is small, easy to access, and situated so that a complete margin of healthy tissue can be taken and analyzed. The *margin* is the border of normal tissue remaining around the tumor that has been removed. A margin that is clear of cancer indicates that the entire tumor has been removed and the chance of cancer returning to the same site is low.

For most early-stage breast cancers, lumpectomy includes biopsy of the lymph nodes to check them for cancer. A lumpectomy is nearly always followed by radiation. The combination of lumpectomy and radiation is

Lumpectomy

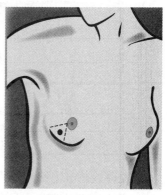

In a lumpectomy procedure, the lump and surrounding tissue are removed.

Quadrantectomy

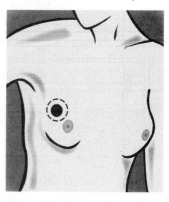

When performing a quadrantectomy, the surgeon removes the tumor, and the quadrant of tissue containing the tumor, and the lining over the chest muscles.

as effective as mastectomy. Most lumpectomies are performed on an outpatient basis.

Quadrantectomy. For a *quadrantectomy,* a surgeon removes most of one quadrant, or about one-fourth of the breast, including the skin and connective tissue and sometimes the underarm lymph nodes. This procedure may be the best choice when a tumor is large or the breast is small. After surgery, the affected breast might be noticeably smaller than the other breast.

Follow-up surgery can equalize breast size and restore symmetry, either by enlarging the smaller breast or reducing the size of the larger one. Oftentimes, the smaller breast can be enlarged with fat grafting—removing fat from another part of the body and inserting it into the breast.

Total Mastectomy

For a *total mastectomy,* a surgeon removes the entire breast; sometimes the nipple can be saved. No axillary lymph nodes are removed. The *axillary lymph nodes* are a group of twenty to thirty lymph nodes located in the deep tissues in and around the armpit. A sentinel node biopsy is performed to check for any cancer cells that have spread to these lymph nodes; a sentinel node biopsy refers to removing only the first one to three lymph nodes in the area of the armpit. (*See* more on sentinel node biopsy in the next section.)

A total mastectomy is often performed when cancer is detected in more than one duct or lobe in the breast. If reconstruction is planned, a surgeon can make efforts to spare skin and the nipple as long as the skin and nipple are free of cancer cells.

A total mastectomy is also an effective *prophylactic* (preventive) procedure for women at high risk for breast cancer as a result of abnormal genes that they have inherited.

Sentinel Node Biopsy

As mentioned in chapter 2, a sentinel node biopsy is performed to determine the possible spread of breast cancer into nearby lymph nodes. The sentinel node in the armpit is usually the first node to which lymph fluid drains from a breast tumor, so it is the first node in which spreading cancer cells are likely to appear. To perform this procedure, the surgeon injects a blue dye, or a radioactive tracer, near the tumor. This substance then shows up clearly on a handheld monitor, making it possible for the surgeon to see the path the dye takes from the tumor to the lymph nodes. The first node reached by the dye is the sentinel node. If cancer is found in the sentinel node, other nodes in the area are removed because they may contain cancer cells as well.

Removing only one node or a few lymph nodes is a less extensive operation compared to removing all or most of the nodes. Further, the sentinel node procedure is considered as reliable as the removal of all the underarm area lymph nodes, and it is much less likely to result in complications such as

Total Mastectomy

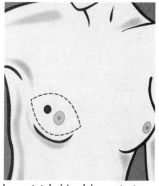

In a total (simple) mastectomy procedure, the entire breast is removed, but no lymph nodes are removed.

Modified Radical Mastectomy

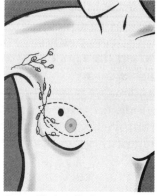

A modified radical mastectomy involves removing the entire breast, and all breast tissue extending toward the breastbone, collarbone, and to the lowest ribs; also lymph nodes in the armpit are removed and sometimes in the minor pectoral muscle.

lymphedema, which is swelling caused by the removal of lymph nodes.

Sentinel node biopsy is usually done at the time of lumpectomy or mastectomy but is sometimes done at the time of breast biopsy or shortly thereafter in patients who are going to receive chemotherapy prior to surgery.

Modified Radical Mastectomy

The *modified radical mastectomy,* an older approach to breast removal and rarely performed today, removes all breast tissue, covering an area from the breastbone to the back of the armpit and from the collarbone to the lower bra line, and some or all of the axillary lymph nodes. Occasionally, the small strap-like pectoralis minor muscle above the breast is removed if it interferes with lymph node removal or if it has been invaded by cancer cells. Today, however, because the vast majority of breast cancers are discovered before they invade the chest muscles, the cancer can be removed using simpler, less invasive surgery.

The modified radical mastectomy is performed when the cancer's size, stage, or location rules out partial mastectomy. Cancers located in several parts of a breast and most stage II and stage III cancers are treated with modified radical mastectomy because the procedure removes not only the breast tissue but also the cancerous lymph nodes.

Postsurgical Drains

Immediately after a mastectomy, a surgeon may place soft plastic tubes, or drains, under the skin near the closed incision. The tubes prevent discomfort and possibly infection by carrying away the tissue fluid that builds up while the incision is healing. You might see some blood in this fluid at first, but it will soon be pale yellow, collecting in a small bulb at the end of each tube. The drains are removed when the fluid diminishes, usually after five to seven days.

Let your doctor know immediately about any severe pain, which could be a sign of internal bleeding or a hematoma, which is blood pooling in tissue at the surgical site.

I had a double mastectomy and was surprised that I had very little pain. Actually, the hardest part for me was losing my hair during chemotherapy.

—*Shirley, 58*

Pain Management

Lumpectomy and mastectomy aren't generally associated with intense postoperative pain; however, managing any pain after breast surgery is essential to your comfort and to the healing process. With discomfort at a minimum, you're better able to get the rest you need to recover.

Several pain management options are available during your hospital stay and during your recovery at home. Depending on your procedure, your postsurgical pain relief options while in the hospital may include pain-relieving drugs, which are delivered through an intravenous line, patient-controlled analgesia (PCA), and the newer "pain relief ball." Pain relievers in pill form may also be given in the hospital or taken later at home.

Intraoperative Pain Management

Today, pain management can actually begin during your surgery. *Intraoperative pain management* delivers anti-inflammatories and acetaminophen through an IV; an injection of a long-acting anesthetic is also given in the breast. This anesthetic blocks the nerves where they enter the chest muscles, providing pain relief for up to three days, in contrast with regular local anesthetic that would give eight hours of relief.

Intraoperative pain management reduces the need for postsurgical narcotics, allows a patient to be up and moving around sooner, and decreases the length of hospital stays. In fact, the anesthetic technique allows some patients to return home the same day as the surgery.

Intravenous (IV) Pain Medication

A common pain management method used in hospitals following breast surgery is intravenous (IV) pain medication. With this method, opioid medications, such as morphine or Dilaudid, are delivered to you through your IV line. A nurse administers the medication at prescribed intervals, approximately every four hours. If you should continue to experience pain, notify your nurse, who may either administer another dose or consult with your surgeon about adjusting the dosage.

Have someone with you before and after your surgery. My eighty-year-old mother was with me and she kept saying she felt so useless because she couldn't do any housework or laundry for me. But she didn't realize what a help she was just by being there. It made a total difference.

—*Marie, 45*

Patient-Controlled Analgesia (PCA)

During a hospital stay, pain relief may be administered through *patient-controlled analgesia (PCA)*. With PCA, pain medications, such as morphine, Demerol, or Dilaudid, are delivered through your intravenous line. The IV line is attached to a computerized pump that is usually mounted on a pole near your bed. When you feel pain, you simply press a button to activate the pump, which delivers a dose of medication. The pump is calibrated so that it is impossible to give yourself too many dosages.

It's usually best to give yourself small, frequent doses of the pain medication to provide steady relief. Waiting until your pain gets worse is not advisable and may make it more difficult for you to get comfortable again.

Opioid Medications

Opioid medications, also called *narcotics* or *opiates,* are commonly taken in pill form and are used to alleviate moderate to severe pain in the days following a mastectomy or lumpectomy. However, many women find that they need the medication for only a few days, if any, following surgery.

Commonly prescribed opioids for use at home include Tylenol with codeine, Vicodin, and Percocet. Although these medications can be habit-forming, they will not lead to addiction when taken, as directed, for short periods of time. The drugs can be obtained only through a physician's prescription. Opioids have side effects, including nausea, sleepiness, constipation, and slowed breathing.

Non-Opioid Medications

Non-opioid pain relievers are non-narcotic, and many of them do not require a doctor's prescription. Designed to control mild to moderate pain, these medications include acetaminophen and nonsteroidal anti-inflammatory drugs (NSAIDs), such as ibuprofen and naproxen. Even though these drugs may not require a prescription, it's important to check with your doctor before taking them. Side effects are rarely associated with acetaminophen when taken for short periods. NSAIDs, however, can cause stomach pain, heartburn, dizziness, and constipation. Inform your doctor if you experience any side effects.

Recovery after Breast Surgery

Once your breast surgery is over, your recovery begins. Recovery from lumpectomy is relatively quick. However, recovery from mastectomy or mastectomy with lymph node removal requires more time, and complete

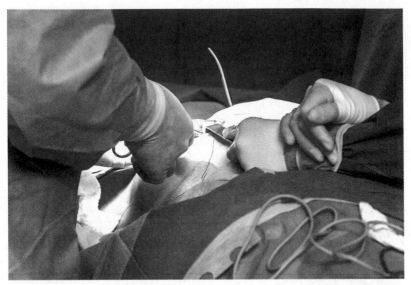

Surgery is a first-line treatment for breast cancer. Some women are able to choose between mastectomy, removal of the entire breast, and lumpectomy, removal of a tumor along with a rim of normal tissue.

recovery may take six to eight weeks. No matter which kind of surgery you've had, you'll notice improvement with each passing day.

If you've had a lumpectomy, you can expect to return to normal activities, such as walking, showering, and driving, within a day or two. Most women feel well enough to return to work within a few days. If you have had a sentinel node biopsy as part of your lumpectomy, it may take a few extra days before you're ready to return to work and other normal activities.

If you've had a mastectomy, it will be a week or more before you're ready to return to normal activities. If you've had a mastectomy with lymph node removal, you're likely to need some assistance with everyday tasks for a few weeks, such as washing your hair or caring for your children.

Following mastectomy with or without lymph node removal, your return to work depends in part on the type of work you do. If you have an office job, you'll be able to return to work sooner than if your work involves heavy lifting or strenuous labor. Some women return to work within a week; others take two or more weeks before going back to work.

Possible Side Effects of Surgery

Hematoma

A *hematoma* is a potential postsurgical complication that occurs when blood pools at the surgery site as a result of a leaking or ruptured blood vessel. Hematomas that occur in the breast after surgery may feel like a lump and may be painful. It is important to report this to your surgeon right away since a hematoma can cause tissue death in the area in which the bleeding occurs.

Anxiety and Depression

Some women are depressed after even the most successful surgery. Your body's response to the trauma of surgery can make you sad or anxious, as can the mental stress of a cancer diagnosis.

If you had a mastectomy, your first look at the place where your breast used to be may be difficult. You might even be a little afraid of seeing the surgery site after the bandages are removed. But putting it off will only create greater anxiety. When the time comes, you might want your partner or close friend there to "hold your hand."

Many women actually aren't as upset over their appearance after having had a breast removed as they expected to be. Relief that the tumor is gone usually outweighs their distress about scarring and even their very natural grief over losing a breast.

Restricted Arm Mobility and Numbness

If your lymph nodes were removed, your arm may be stiff for a few days to a few weeks. Physical therapy can help. You'll probably be shown some easy stretching and pulling exercises that will immediately improve your mobility. Eventually you'll have full, normal use of your arm. Even if small portions of muscle have been removed, your strength will return. During lymph node removal, a nerve may have been cut. This is normal and not a cause for worry, though it can cause some unpleasant symptoms. Your upper arm might be numb, and starting a few days after the operation, you may feel tingling, sharp pains, or squeezing pressure. These sensations will go away in a week or two, although in a few cases (2 to 3 percent) a chronic ache remains.

Phantom Breast

Up to 80 percent of women who have had a mastectomy report that they can "feel" the missing breast, much as people "feel" a limb that has been amputated. If your breast tumor was painful, you might feel the "ghost" of that pain for weeks or months after your surgery. Some women have "phantom breast" sensations on and off for years—not painful, simply there. These sensations are being recalled by the brain, which does not forget. They do not mean the cancer has returned. Nevertheless, it is important to check with your doctor if any new or unusual pain begins, one that has not already been identified as a phantom sensation.

Lymphedema

If your arm should become inflamed—brought on by anything from a mosquito bite to a strained muscle—your body sends extra lymph fluid, which carries infection-fighting white blood cells, to the site of the inflammation. But if the lymph nodes and vessels have been removed from that side of your body, they're no longer available to drain away excess lymph. With nowhere to go, the fluid collects in your arm, causing it to swell.

Tips for Preventing Lymphedema

- Lift nothing heavier than ten pounds with the affected arm while you're healing.

- Any exercise program or physical activity involving the arm should begin gradually and include frequent rest breaks.

- Get in the habit of consistent low-impact exercise, such as walking, swimming, or stretching.

- Don't carry a heavy purse over the affected shoulder.

- Be very protective of the affected arm to avoid injury that could lead to infection. Keep it clean. Use sunscreen and insect repellent. Use moisturizer to avoid chapping and cuticle cream to avoid hangnails (and don't cut your cuticles). Use an electric shaver, not a razor, to shave your underarms; don't use chemical hair removers. Protect your hands and arms when cooking or taking food out of a hot oven. Wear protective gloves for gardening and yard work, and rubber gloves when you're cleaning with chemicals and doing the dishes.

- Ask medical personnel not to use the affected arm to take your blood pressure, draw blood, or give an injection.

- If you get even a tiny cut or puncture, wash it with soap and water, apply an antibacterial ointment, and keep an eye on it for signs of infection.

- If you plan to take a long trip by air, consider wearing a compression garment to keep swelling down. Compression garments are sold online, in mail-order catalogs, and at many pharmacies. If you need a professionally fitted or custom-fitted compression garment, ask your doctor where you can obtain one in your area.

- Ask your doctor or a physical therapist for post-mastectomy exercises you can do to reduce the risk of lymphedema.

This condition, called lymphedema, occurs in up to 20 percent of women who have had axillary dissection. The risk of lymphedema is lowest with sentinel node biopsy and highest with complete axillary dissection.

Lymphedema is not life-threatening, but it can be painful and needs prompt treatment. If the symptoms are ignored, the fluid can become infected and, in severe cases, there can be permanent damage to the arm.

Because you can develop lymphedema anytime, even years after your surgery, you may need to make prevention a lifelong regimen. This means maintaining a healthy weight and avoiding injury, infection, constriction, muscle strain, and temperature extremes, starting immediately after your surgery.

See your doctor right away if you have swelling or pain in your arm; if an injury becomes puffy or tender; if your skin feels hot or is inflamed in any way—a rash, itching, or redness—;or if you have a fever or flu-like symptoms. Antibiotics and diuretics, given early on, can help, as can physical therapy and specialized massages given by a lymphedema therapist.

For more information about lymphedema, contact the National Lymphedema Network, listed in the Resources section at the back of this book.

Infection

If you notice even a slight swelling of your affected arm soon after mastectomy, or if swelling, redness, or warmth occurs under the incision, it could be a sign of infection. Notify your doctor immediately. Such infections can be serious and should be treated without delay.

Postsurgical Prognosis

After your surgery, when the pathologist has examined the tumor and other tissues that were removed, your doctor will have a better idea about the need for additional treatment. The best possible news would be that the entire tumor and a clear margin have been removed, lymph node analysis shows no cancer cells, and you can expect a full recovery.

The majority of women with breast cancer are cured. Even so, you'll need close follow-up, since not even the best outcome can guarantee that every cancer cell is gone or that cancer will not return. Getting rid of remaining cancer after surgery is the purpose of *adjuvant therapy*—treatment given after the primary treatment (surgery, in this case) to improve the chance for a cure. Adjuvant therapy may be *local*—for example, radiation directed at the cancer site—or *systemic,* affecting the entire body, as with chemotherapy and hormone-blocking and targeted therapies.

If lymph nodes removed during surgery test positive for cancer or if your cancer was of a comparatively rare type that has a high risk of recurrence, your doctor will prescribe one or more forms of adjuvant therapy. If your tumor was node-negative (that is, with no cancer found in the lymph nodes), the doctor will probably order more tests to find out if you could benefit from adjuvant therapies as protection against recurrence.

Your prognosis depends on many factors, including your overall health, your individual anatomy, and your responses to therapy. Thus, your doctors will not be able to guarantee a particular prognosis. At best, they can tell you about general patterns of recovery, or recurrence, in cases similar to yours.

However, no two cases are exactly alike. Many women meet bad news with a positive attitude and live longer than their prognosis seemed to predict. Meanwhile, new discoveries and treatments continually emerge, lengthening lives and instantly making older statistics obsolete. Continuing developments in therapy hold great promise for breast cancer patients.

5

Breast Reconstruction

It has been said that "mastectomy treats the disease and reconstruction heals the mind." For women with breast cancer, treating the disease is the first and by far the most important consideration. Today, breast reconstruction is often a close second. You may be among the many women who, though forever grateful for the recovery from breast cancer, welcome the possibility of restoring the appearance of a natural breast in place of the one that was lost.

When performed by a properly trained and experienced plastic surgeon, breast reconstruction is a safe and effective option for almost any woman who has had a breast removed. In many cases, it can be done either at the time of the original breast surgery or later, even years later.

In larger hospitals throughout the country, breast cancer is often treated with a comprehensive team approach. The team normally includes a mastectomy surgeon, a reconstruction surgeon, physicians who specialize in chemotherapy and radiation, and other support personnel. This team approach is ideal because it allows for close communication among all of the team members participating in your care. It is important that the technique and timing of your reconstruction is coordinated with the mastectomy and any chemotherapy or radiation therapy that might be necessary.

Breast Reconstruction or External Prostheses?

The choice to have breast reconstruction is intensely personal. Many women feel strong, confident, and content without reconstruction. The choice often depends on lifestyle, fashion preferences, and personal preference.

Some women choose to utilize an external prosthesis. This is an excellent option for women who can't have or don't want reconstruction. Today's prostheses are lighter and less bulky than the older types, and you can start wearing them when you have healed sufficiently, often as soon as six weeks after your mastectomy. The prosthesis materials may be made of silicone gel or fiberfill. Often, they are made to fit into the pockets of post-mastectomy bras; others adhere directly to the chest.

I kept a journal through my breast cancer experience to remember things so I could help others. The day of my surgery, I gave my journal to my friends and family who were with me in the hospital, and they wrote their thoughts. Those have been the pages I have read the most.

—Marilyn, 61

However, most women who choose reconstruction are concerned more about the way they look when they are not fully clothed. Their breasts are often important to their sexuality, confidence, and sense of femininity. They want to feel whole as well as look whole—they want to shower, dress, walk, reach, and bend with two breasts in place. For some women, the mastectomy scar can be an ever-present reminder of the cancer. Breast reconstruction is often successful in removing the constant reminder of the mastectomy experience.

Breast Reconstruction Plan

By performing a breast reconstruction procedure, the surgeon creates a breast mound that is as natural-looking as possible. The goal of breast reconstruction is to restore

Breast Implant

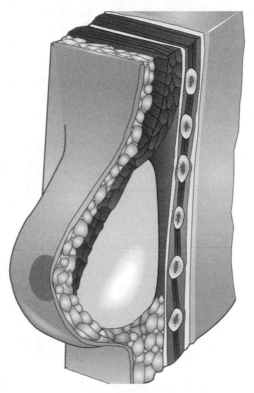

An implant is the most common method of breast reconstruction. Typically, a tissue expander, filled gradually with saline, is used to stretch the skin so it will accommodate the insertion of an implant.

form and symmetry (evenness) to the chest wall. If only one breast is reconstructed, no matter how realistic it is, it won't look exactly like a natural breast. Thus, many women choose to modify the opposite natural breast with an implant, breast reduction, or breast lift so that it most closely resembles the reconstructed breast.

Request for removal of both breasts has steadily increased over the last several years. In addition to reducing future risk, it has been shown that there is a higher degree of patient satisfaction when both breasts are removed at the same time and followed by reconstruction. This is in contrast to women who choose unilateral (one-sided) mastectomy and unilateral reconstruction

Breast reconstruction should never be allowed to interfere with the main priority—eliminating the cancer. Fortunately, with the new team approach to the management of breast cancer, the timing and technique of your reconstructive surgery can be scheduled to optimally fit into the overall plan, which may include radiation and/or chemotherapy.

Immediate or Delayed Reconstruction?

After consulting with members of your breast cancer team, you can make a decision about whether or not your reconstruction is performed, or at least started, at the time of your mastectomy. If you are undecided you can opt to undergo delayed reconstruction at a later time.

Advantages of Immediate Reconstruction

- *Financial.* It normally costs less to have the mastectomy and the reconstruction performed at the same time.
- *Emotional-Psychological.* Immediate reconstruction often eliminates or reduces two sources of distress—a second surgery later on, and the experience of waking up from the first surgery with no breast whatsoever.
- *Personal choice.* Some women who would be candidates for a lumpectomy with subsequent radiation choose instead to have a mastectomy with immediate reconstruction in order to avoid the radiation.
- *Practical considerations.* Women with jobs outside the home can minimize their time away from work by consolidating the surgeries. Stay-at-home

mothers won't have to arrange child care around two operations.

- *Cosmetic factors.* In many cases, immediate reconstruction leads to a better cosmetic result.

Reasons for Delayed Reconstruction

- *Further treatment needed.* If radiation is required, it is sometimes best to delay the reconstruction.
- *Advanced breast cancer.* Having advanced cancer may be a reason to postpone the procedure.
- *Overall health.* If overall general health is poor or if a patient is suffering emotional problems, it is probably best to delay the procedure. For example, the best time to have reconstructive surgery is not when you are in the middle of a financial crisis, a divorce, or bereavement.
- *Time to collect information.* Delaying reconstruction gives you time to think about your options and become informed. The decision-making process for breast surgery alone can be overwhelming. By putting off reconstruction, you can weigh your options carefully, recover from your mastectomy, and find out whether you even want or need reconstruction.

Reconstruction Options

Options for breast reconstruction continue to improve. With every option, it is important to weigh the advantages and disadvantages of the procedure, recovery, and long-term results. Whichever technique is utilized, the opposite breast is usually modified for the sake of a balanced appearance; this may mean a breast lift, a breast reduction, or breast augmentation. In some cases, it may mean removing and reconstructing the opposite breast. More and more women are choosing double mastectomies in order to reduce future risk and provide for a better overall aesthetic outcome.

Reconstruction with Implants

The majority of women undergoing breast reconstruction today choose to have breast implants. The benefits of implant reconstruction include shorter recovery times and less invasive surgical procedures.

One-stage procedure. In some cases, breast implant reconstruction can be performed as a single-stage procedure with an implant being placed at the time of the mastectomy. This is particularly true for the increased number of women who have opted for nipple-sparing mastectomies. In a nipple-sparing mastectomy, the nipple and surrounding areola are not removed. This approach maintains an intact skin "envelope" (where the implant will be inserted) which can allow for immediate reconstruction with only the implant. In this procedure, the implant is placed under the chest muscle.

During implant reconstruction, I was uncomfortable sleeping on my stomach and on my side. I learned to prop up pillows at my back and under my arm to sleep more comfortably.

—*Suzanne, 58*

Direct-to-implant reconstruction. Within the last several years there has been a steady increase in a procedure called *direct-to-implant reconstruction.* In this procedure, the nipple and areola is spared and a permanent implant is placed into the skin envelope remaining after the mastectomy. However, this procedure differs from the traditional one-stage procedure in that the implant is placed on top of the chest muscle. (The reason for placing the implant under the muscle was to provide thicker tissue coverage over the implant.) But as mastectomy techniques have improved, it is the standard to leave thicker skin flaps. Placing the implant over the muscle leads to easier recovery. If a thicker flap is needed over the implant, the surgeon can use fat grafting or other materials to create additional tissue coverage over the implant.

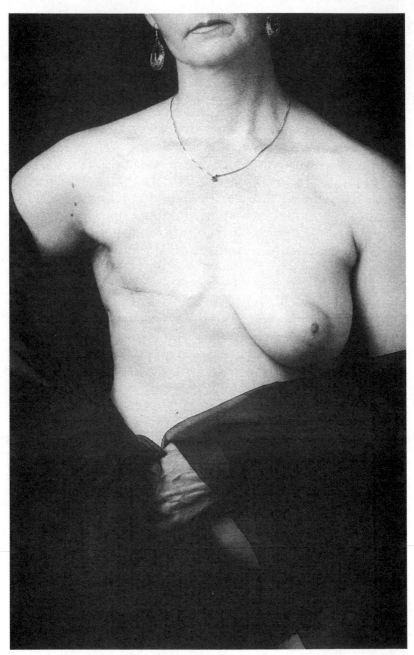

This woman had a mastectomy at age forty-three.

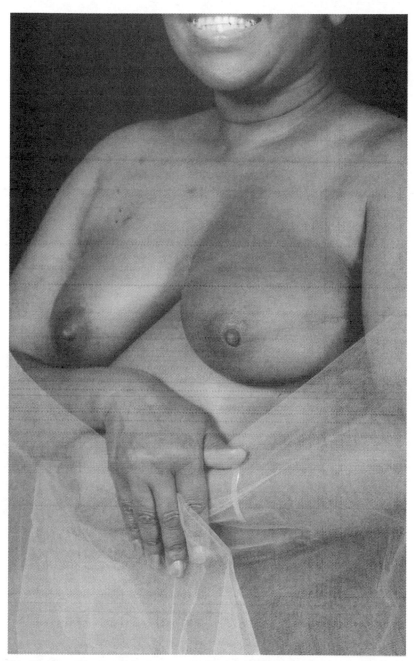

This fifty-year-old woman's breast cancer in her left breast was detected early. She had a lumpectomy, in which the cancerous growth and surrounding tissue were removed.

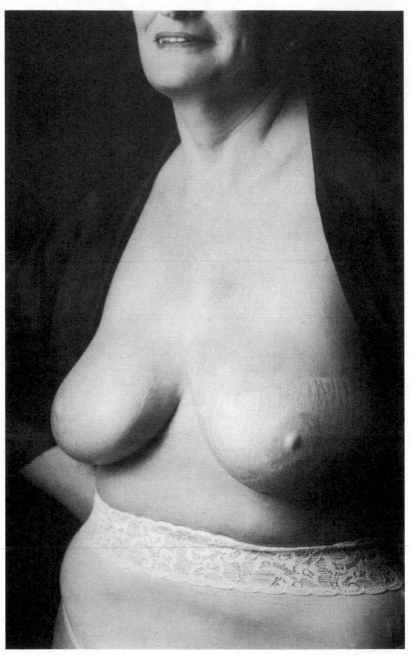

At age forty-seven, this woman had both breasts removed. She chose a bilateral (both sides) TRAM flap reconstruction, followed by reconstruction of the nipple and areola.

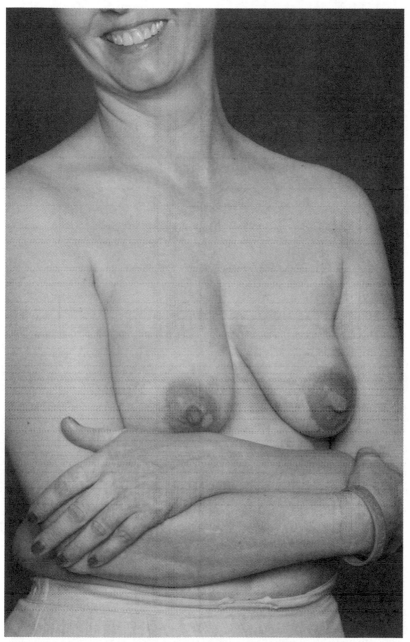

This woman was forty-three-years old when diagnosed with breast cancer in her left breast. She underwent a lumpectomy, which was followed by radiation therapy. Her scar, on the right side of her left breast, is barely visible.

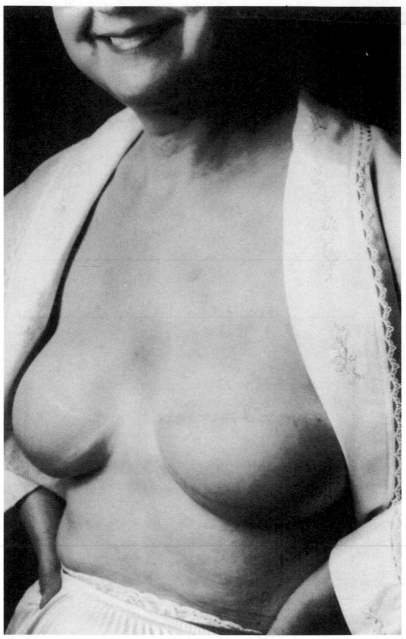

At age fifty, this woman had a bilateral mastectomy. She chose to have saline implants and is not planning to have nipple and areola reconstruction.

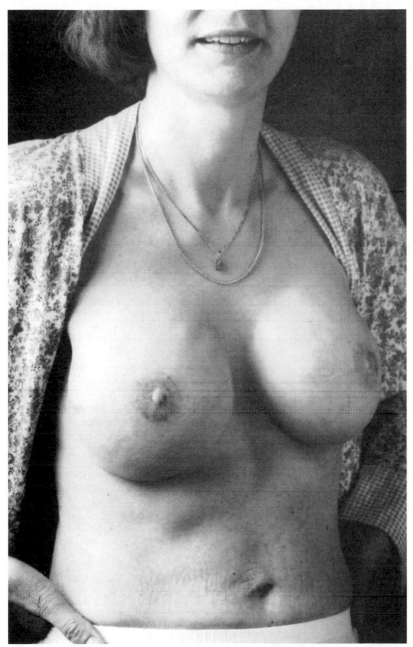

This woman, age thirty-eight at the time of her surgery, had both breasts removed. She chose to have tissue expanders with saline implants. During a second procedure, she had nipple and areola reconstruction.

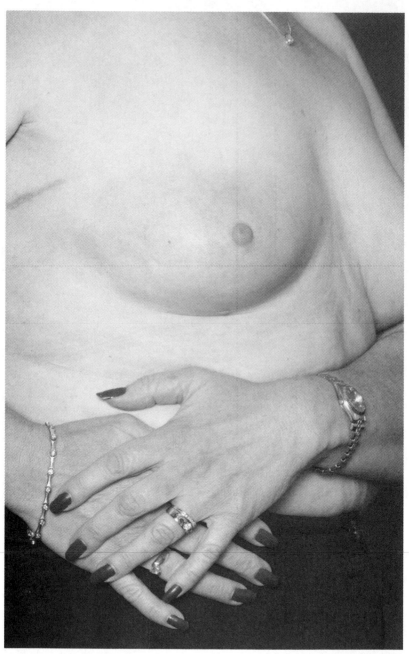

At age forty-nine, this woman chose to have a lumpectomy performed on her right breast. She also underwent six weeks of radiation therapy.

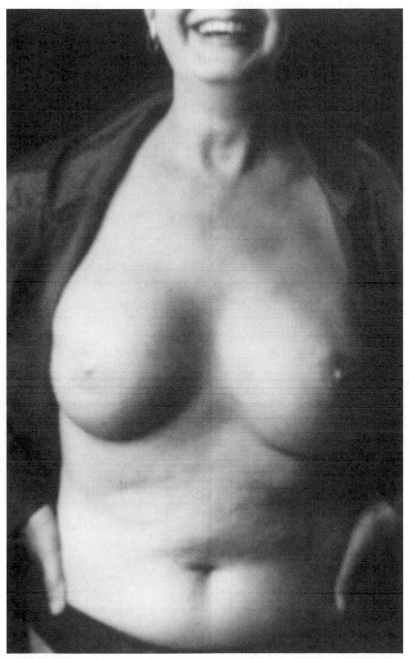

Tissue expanders were inserted immediately following this forty-six-year-old woman's double mastectomy. Saline implants were placed six weeks later, followed by reconstruction of the nipple and areola.

The direct-to-implant procedure requires planning between the mastectomy surgeon and the reconstructive surgeon.

Two-Stage Procedure. In many cases, reconstruction with an implant is a two-stage process. The first stage involves placement of a device called a *tissue expander* at the time of the mastectomy. The tissue expander can be placed either in the skin pocket remaining after the mastectomy or under the chest wall muscle. This decision will be made by the reconstructive surgeon at the time of the mastectomy. Over several weeks, sterile saline is injected into the tissue expander, gradually stretching the tissues to create a pocket. After a satisfactory pocket has been developed, the expander is removed and an implant is inserted.

Fat Grafting

There have been significant improvements in the process and efficacy of fat grafting in recent years. The process of fat grafting involves removing fat from a different part of the body and injecting it into the area of the breast. This procedure has become a useful addition to the process of implant reconstruction.

The technique of fat grafting has improved over the last several years, mostly because there is a better understanding of how to remove and reinject the fat, combined with newer processes to prepare the fat for injection after it is removed from a different part of the body.

Types of Breast Implants

The implants utilized for breast reconstruction consist of a silicone shell filled with either saline or silicone gel. Silicone and saline are considered equally safe. Both saline and silicone implants come in different shapes and sizes. Both have several variations of round designs.

Saline-filled Implants

Saline is salt water. It is the same type of fluid used in intravenous (IV) therapy. Consequently it is compatible with the human body if it should leak.

Silicone-filled Implants

Silicone gel is a much thicker substance than saline but is considered to be more like a natural breast to the touch. Normally when silicone gel leaks it stays within the pocket the body has created around the implant. Silicone implants were approved as being safe and effective by the FDA in 2006. Silicone implants come in contoured or "teardrop" shapes. A teardrop implant is less full in the upper portion, and it tapers out to a fuller lower portion. A teardrop implant has a textured outer surface to keep it from rotating.

Potential Complications with Breast Implants

Breast implant reconstruction has a range of potential complications. The following are the among the most common complications.

Wrinkling

One of the problems with breast implants has been visible wrinkling. All implants have some degree of wrinkling. Normally, wrinkling is seen when the soft tissue coverage over the implant is thin. There have been advances in the prevention of wrinkling. These include improved techniques, fat grafting, and newer types of implants that contain a thicker gel and are highly cohesive. The more cohesive material feels like a gummy bear candy and is less likely to show wrinkling.

Capsular Contracture

The body will naturally form a lining around the implant. This lining is called a *capsule*. The formation of the capsule is normal and expected. Very likely the formation of the capsule is the body's way of walling itself off from a foreign object. In some cases this lining can thicken and actually shrink and compress the implant. This is called a *capsular contracture*. It will cause the implant to feel unnaturally firm.

If this complication occurs, the repair may involve removal of the thickened capsule or possibly creating several incisions in the capsule to allow it to expand. Patients may be prescribed steroid and anti-inflammatory drugs for several weeks after the release of the capsule contracture to help prevent recurrence of this complication.

Infection

Although infection rates are low they do sometimes occur. If the pocket containing the expander or the implant becomes infected it is normally necessarily to temporarily remove the device and wait for adequate healing before proceeding further.

Leakage

With leakage in a saline breast implant, the breast changes shape rapidly as the saltwater fluid leaks out. This causes a cosmetic change, but it is not dangerous because saline is compatible with the human body if it should leak.

Leakage that occurs in a silicone implant occurs slowly. Signs of a ruptured implant may include changes in breast shape and size, firmness, increasing pain, and swelling over a period of weeks. Silicone implant rupture that doesn't cause any noticeable symptoms is known as a silent rupture.

To diagnose the problem, a surgeon may ask you to undergo ultrasound testing, a mammogram, or an MRI to determine whether the implant has ruptured. Although the ruptured implant does not represent a health hazard, most surgeons recommend removing the implant and replacing it with a new one.

Breast Implant Syndrome

In 2019, the Food and Drug Administration identified a possible association between breast implants and a rare cancer of the immune system—breast implant–associated anaplastic large cell lymphoma (BIA-ALCL). The FDA states that women with breast implants that have textured surfaces have a very low but increased risk of developing the cancer. Further research is ongoing to examine the relationship between the cancer and breast implants.

Symptoms may include pain near an implant, fluid collection around the implant, fatigue, fever, dry eyes, dry mouth, muscle ache, and trouble concentrating. To date, 467 cases of anaplastic large cell lymphoma have been diagnosed worldwide. The treatment—removal of the surrounding capsule—normally cures the condition.

Extrusion

This is rare, but occasionally the overlying tissue breaks down and the implant or the expander becomes visible. This will require removal of the device and very likely secondary surgery utilizing your own tissue for reconstruction.

Reconstruction with Your Own Tissue

When your own tissue is used for reconstruction, it is called *autologous reconstruction*. Autologous reconstruction is accomplished by transferring a "flap" of your own tissue into the area to be reconstructed. A *flap* refers to transferring tissue that is still connected to a blood supply. This is in contrast to a graft. A *graft* refers to tissue that is removed from one part of the body and placed in another part of the body, anticipating that the body will grow a blood supply into it and keep it alive.

TRAM Flap

The hallmark flap procedure for autologous reconstruction has always been the *TRAM flap*. TRAM is an abbreviation for the *transverse rectus abdominis myocutaneous* flap. In a TRAM flap procedure, the skin and fat of the lower part of the abdomen are transferred to the chest wall to reconstruct the missing breast. It is possible to transfer the flap of skin by keeping it attached to its blood supply.

In this procedure, a flap of skin and fat from the belly button down to the pubic bone and across the abdomen from hip to hip, is separated from all of its attachments; however, this flap stays attached to the lower part of the *rectus muscle.* Also known as the *abdominal muscle,* the rectus muscle is a long, narrow muscle extending from the rib cage down to the pubic bone. There are two rectus muscles, one on each side of the abdomen.

The rectus muscle, along with the attached skin and fat of the lower abdomen, is then lifted upward out of its bed up to the rib cage. The tissue of the lower abdomen, while still remaining attached to the rectus muscle, is transferred through a tunnel up to the chest wall and the tissue is then molded and shaped to reconstruct the breast.

The blood supply to the transferred skin and fat is maintained through the blood flow in the rectus muscle. Because abdominal fat and breast tissue are about the same consistency, the new breast usually looks and feels quite natural. As a bonus, the patient gets a flatter abdomen since the tissues used are those removed during a "tummy tuck."

TRAM flap surgery is much more extensive than implant surgery, requiring between three to five hours for the procedure. A hospital stay of two to four nights is usually required, followed by eight to twelve weeks for full recovery.

If your procedure is performed by an experienced surgeon the complication rate should be low. However, potential complications include lack of sufficient blood supply to the flap, causing complete or partial loss of the tissue, infection, and a possible abdominal wall hernia.

TRAM Flap

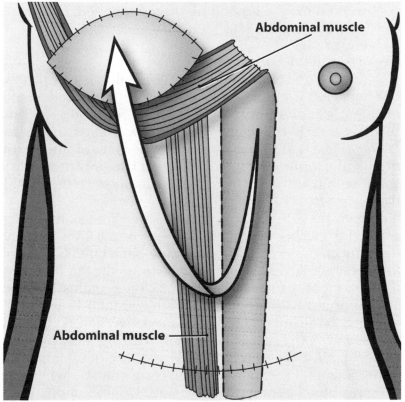

During a TRAM flap procedure, skin, fat, and muscle from the lower abdomen are used. The abdominal muscle is disconnected, but left anchored to the rib cage. Then the skin and fat, which remain attached to the muscle, are rotated upward to form the breast. The fat tissue in the flap helps form the new breast.

You may not be a good candidate for a TRAM flap if:

- You are obese or very thin.
- You have abdominal scars from a previous surgery that may have interrupted the blood supply to the tissue required.
- You are a smoker. Smoking diminishes the blood supply to the skin and fat of the lower abdomen. This can lead to loss of the transferred tissue and wound healing problems in the lower abdomen.

- You have diabetes or other blood vessel disease.
- You have heart or lung disease or are in otherwise poor health.

Free Flap Reconstruction

A *free flap* refers to a flap of tissue that is completely disconnected from the body. It is then transferred to the recipient site and the blood supply is reconnected. This blood vessel is called the *deep inferior epigastric vessel (DIEP)*. The DIEP flap has become one of the most frequently performed procedures that use only the body's tissue to reconstruct a breast. It is variation of the TRAM flap.

With the DIEP flap technique, the same skin and fat of the lower abdomen that are used in a TRAM flap are disconnected from all surrounding attachments except for one blood vessel that travels from the groin up to the bottom of the rectus muscle (abdominal muscle). The skin and fat of the lower abdomen are then brought up to the chest wall and the blood vessel is then reattached to a blood vessel in the chest wall, utilizing a microscope to accomplish the attachment. This technique eliminates requirement for the transfer of the rectus muscle while still keeping blood supply to the tissue. Complications such as abdominal wall hernia are less likely in this technique.

Gluteal Flap Reconstruction

Another reconstruction method uses free flaps taken from the gluteal area called the *SGAP flap (superior gluteal artery perforator flap)* or *IGAP flap (inferior gluteal artery perforator flap)*. These methods use skin, fat, and muscle from the upper or lower portion of the buttock. In these procedures, a wedge from one of the buttocks is transferred and shaped to form the new breast. A microscope is required to reattach the blood vessel to a recipient vessel on the chest wall. These procedures are

Latissimus Dorsi Flap Reconstruction

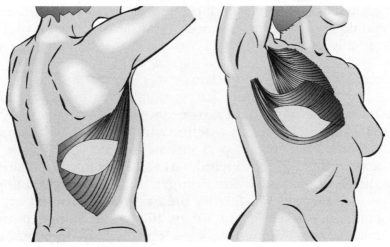

In this procedure, the latissimus dorsi muscle in the back is disconnected, but stays attached at the armpit. The skin and fat, attached to the muscle, are pulled around to form the breast. This procedure usually also requires an implant for volume.

longer and more complicated than other flap procedures and are not frequently performed.

The free flap procedures which include the DIEP flap, the SGAP flap, and the IGAP flap require a highly skilled team for optimal performance and normally require considerably longer times in the operating room. Consequently, these procedures are usually only offered in larger hospitals or teaching institutions.

Latissimus Dorsi Muscle Flap Reconstruction.

The latissimus dorsi muscle is a broad flat muscle in the middle of the back. Divided into two segments along the spine, the latissimus muscles are commonly referred to as "lats." In this procedure, an oval flap made up of a section of this muscle, skin, and fat, is pulled around to the chest to form the breast. The flap stays attached at the armpit, allowing all the blood vessels and arteries to stay intact.

A breast implant is often added to create volume. This technique is dependable and is a commonly used technique for reconstruction. Transferring the muscle normally does not affect day-to-day or sporting activities.

Oncoplastic Breast Reconstruction

Oncoplastic refers to surgical techniques that combine the removal of part of the breast (lumpectomy) with immediate reconstruction. In women with large breasts it may mean performing a precisely planned breast reduction that includes the cancer in the portion removed followed by rearrangement of the remaining tissue to create a satisfactory breast form. In women with smaller breasts it might mean filling the lumpectomy cavity with a latissimus dorsi muscle flap transferred from the back. Oncoplastic techniques require very close coordination between the oncologic and reconstructive surgeons and the pathologist responsible for making sure all of the tumor is removed. Because of the highly specialized nature of the techniques, this procedure is not always available.

I was able to get through my reconstruction by telling myself, "You can do this. You're going to look great when it's over!"
—*Joan, 47*

Nipple Areolar Reconstruction

Often, nipple areolar reconstruction is delayed until complete healing of the breast mound reconstruction is achieved. Fortunately there are several good techniques available to reconstruct a natural-appearing nipple areolar complex.

Newer techniques in nipple and areolar tattooing are also available. These include three-dimension (3-D) nipple tattooing. The 3-D tattoos can be quite real looking. The tattoo is actually flat, yet the tattoo artist can give it a three-dimensional look. The tattoos are permanent, but may be touched up over the years if the color fades.

Pain Management after Reconstruction

Breast reconstruction is generally associated with more pain than one might experience with lumpectomy or mastectomy, but any discomfort you may feel can be alleviated with medication. The same pain management options used following a mastectomy are used to minimize postoperative pain after breast reconstruction. These options include opioids—which may be administered intravenously, through a "pain pump," or in pill form.

If you're like most women and require a brief hospital stay following breast reconstruction, opioid pain relievers are likely to be administered during this time. Doctors may prescribe opioids in tapering doses for an additional period of time once you return home. You may switch to over-the-counter, non-opioid pain relievers as soon as you feel ready.

Talk to your surgeon prior to your surgery about how your pain will be managed. It's important to have this matter clarified before you enter the operating room.

Recovery after Reconstruction

Recovery will depend on the type of procedure performed. In procedures utilizing tissue expanders or implants, patients normally have an overnight stay or are treated as an outpatient. Patients are usually back to normal day-to-day activities, including driving a car, in five to seven days. Full recovery usually takes six to eight weeks. Women undergoing a TRAM flap normally have a hospital stay of two to four days. This is usually followed by two weeks at home and then a slow introduction to normal activities such as driving a car. Full recovery is normally eight to twelve weeks.

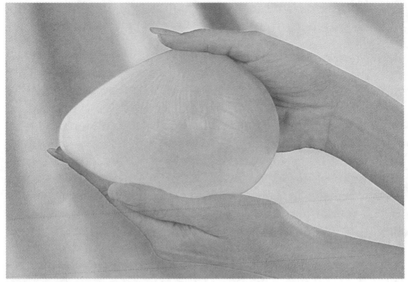

A breast prothesis is made with silicone gel.
Photo courtesy of Amoena.

Prostheses or Breast Forms

If you decide not to have reconstruction, you can always wear a prosthesis. Many women forgo prostheses as well as reconstruction, for any of a number of reasons: They feel no need to conceal the fact that they've had breast surgery, or they're small-breasted to start with, or they like to wear loose clothing, or they just don't want to be bothered with finding, fitting, and wearing an artificial breast.

It's your call. There are as many ways for a woman to feel and look comfortable and confident as there are women.

If you're at your best in tailored, well-fitting clothes, there is no need to sacrifice the look you want. Your surgeon or hospital can put you in touch with a volunteer who is knowledgeable about the numerous and attractive styles of breast prostheses. Some are quite economical and look as good as the pricey ones. The cost can vary widely and is often covered by insurance.

Today's breast forms are not only more convenient and comfortable than older ones but can also be matched to your other breast in size, weight, and appearance. Some attach to the chest wall with the help of a small piece of Velcro-like fabric that can remain painlessly in place for several days or weeks. Others can be secured inside a bra. There are special prostheses for swimming or sports, as well as swimsuits and other garments designed for women who have had mastectomies.

You'll find breast prostheses in catalogs, on the Internet, or in specialized lingerie shops, where you can be fitted for one that is precisely the right size and shape for you.

6

RADIATION THERAPY

Radiation therapy is often prescribed as a follow-up treatment to surgery for breast cancer. Statistics show that radiation therapy can substantially reduce the risk of local recurrence. Cells that are damaged by radiation therapy lose their ability to reproduce, making radiation effective against fast-growing cancer cells. Healthy tissues may also be damaged during treatment; however, the healthy cells heal while the cancer cells do not. Radiation therapy is usually quite tolerable for most women.

Your Radiation Oncologist

A *radiation oncologist* is a physician who specializes in radiation therapy for cancer patients. Most likely, your surgeon or another physician will refer you to this specialist. The initial consultation is an opportunity for you to discuss treatment benefits and risks with the radiation oncologist, who in all likelihood is someone your referring doctor has worked with many times. You are under no obligation to choose this oncologist, and it is your prerogative to ask for another referral.

Consider having a partner, relative, or friend go with you to at least the first meeting with the radiation oncologist—to take notes or ask questions you might forget to ask. Write down as many questions as you can think of in advance. Here are examples of the kinds of things you'll probably be wondering about.

- Will radiation improve my prognosis? To what extent?
- How many treatments will I need? How often will they be given, and for how long?
- Which area will be targeted?
- How much healthy tissue will be exposed to radiation, and where?
- What side effects should I expect, and how can I manage them?

If you live in a rural area or small town, find out where the nearest qualified radiation facility is located. Ask your surgeon or contact the Cancer Information Service of the National Cancer Institute. (*see* the Resources section at the back of this book).

Don't rule out radiation if you live too far from a radiation facility to commute every day. If you don't have friends or relatives who live near a facility and can offer you a place to stay, and you can't afford to stay six weeks or more in a hotel, contact the radiation facility's social worker or patient-support representative. Many medical centers employ people whose job it is to help out with everything from lodging and transportation to financial and family counseling. Programs such as the American Cancer Society's Hope Lodges provide not only free temporary housing during cancer treatment but also a supportive, homelike environment.

A diagnostic test, described in chapter 2, may also be helpful in determining whether you will benefit from radiation therapy (or chemotherapy). You may recall, the Oncotype DX test examines the activity of twenty-one genes and indicates whether the cancer is likely to recur.

You will be a candidate for an Oncotype DX test if:

- you've recently been diagnosed with stage I or II invasive breast cancer
- the cancer is estrogen-receptor-positive
- there is no cancer in your lymph nodes (lymph node-negative breast cancer)
- you and your doctor are making decisions about radiation (or chemotherapy)

Talk to your physician about any of these factors that apply to you.

For stage 0, also known as *DCIS,* a second type of Oncotype DX test can influence the decision as to whether follow-up radiation will be beneficial. As you'll recall from chapter 2, DCIS, or ductal carcinoma *in situ,* is breast cancer of the lining of the milk duct that has not spread outside the milk ducts.

When Is Radiation Used?

After Lumpectomy

Radiation therapy after lumpectomy destroys random cancer cells that might remain in the breast or lymph nodes even when the entire tumor, a clean margin, and any of the lymph nodes have been removed. With standard external beam radiation discussed later in this chapter, the entire breast area is treated by radiation after lumpectomy, including the site from which the tumor was removed. Occassionally, partial breast irradiation that treats the lumpectomy cavity but not the entire breast is appropriate.

After Mastectomy

When the entire breast has been removed and no remaining cancer is detected, radiation is usually unnecessary. If the tumor was large, however, or if cancer was found in the margins or in several lymph nodes, radiation is advisable as a safeguard in case surgery did not remove all the cancer cells.

Similarly, if a large amount of cancer has been removed from the inner breast (near the breastbone) or has been found in several underarm nodes, radiation may be used to treat the lymph nodes behind the breastbone and above the collarbone, since these lymph nodes might also contain cancer cells.

Finally, when a large tumor, five centimeters (two inches) or more, has been shrunk by chemotherapy or hormone-blocking therapy before surgery, radiation after the surgery can reduce the risk of local recurrence.

Radiation was not a bad experience. I actually came to enjoy going every day. In fact, I cried on my last visit because everyone there was so wonderful to me.

—*Sandy, 44*

Delivery of Radiation Therapy

Radiation therapy may be delivered in one of two ways. The standard form of radiation therapy involves delivery of radiation externally—called *external beam radiation.* This form of treatment may be used after mastectomy; it can also be used after a lumpectomy.

The second approach, which may be used after a lumpectomy, is referred to as *brachytherapy.* This form of radiation is delivered internally to the lumpectomy cavity through tiny tubes that are inserted into the breast.

Simulation Appointment

If you are to receive external beam radiation, you'll undergo what's called a *simulation appointment* with your radiation oncologist and his or her team prior to your first treatment. This is a planning session during which the team will determine the precise area to receive the radiation treatment. This plan will be followed carefully during each treatment.

External Beam Radiation

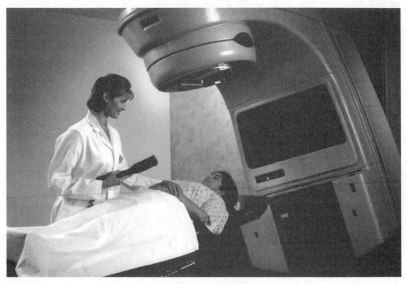

A patient receiving an external beam radiation treatment.
Photo courtesy of Siemens Medical Systems, Inc.

During the simulation, a customized mold will be made for your arm, back, and neck. This mold will be used during your treatments to hold your upper body in place and will reproduce the same position for each treatment.

Part of the simulation appointment will also involve the application of some tiny tattoos—black dots about the size of a pinhead—on your chest to indicate the area to be treated. Most women do not find these tattoos to be cosmetically bothersome; however, they can be removed professionally afterward with a laser.

After the simulation is completed, you'll be scheduled for your first radiation treatment.

External Beam Radiation Therapy

External radiation for cancer treatment reaches its target in the form of a radiation beam, delivered by a machine called a *linear accelerator*. The treatments are painless, much like having an X-ray.

External beam radiation treatments, including preparation, last about ten minutes. A typical treatment schedule is Monday through Friday for three and a half to seven weeks. You're asked not to wear deodorants, powders, creams, lotions, or fragrances when you go to the treatment center. Upon arriving, you'll remove your clothes from the waist up and change into a gown. You'll soon become familiar with the treatment routine.

A specially trained radiation therapist will deliver your treatments. For an external beam radiation treatment, the therapist will usually have you lie on your back; however, some women receive the treatment lying on their abdomen. You'll be asked to lie perfectly still. The radiation machine, which will be above you, will deliver radiation to the tattooed area. The machine will be rotated above you and carefully positioned in two or more places during a treatment session.

Accelerated Breast Radiation Therapy

Some treatment centers are working to shorten the length of time during which whole breast, external beam radiation therapy is given. For example, some doctors are delivering higher doses of radiation over a span of three weeks instead of the typical period of up to seven weeks. This accelerated approach is called *hypofractionated radiation therapy*.

Boost Treatments

Your initial radiation therapy might be followed immediately by boost treatments that zero in on the site from which the tumor was removed. Whether you receive this "boost" dose of radiation will depend on factors such as age, the size and type of your tumor, the width of the margins, and the size of your breast.

Studies show that boost treatments further reduce the risk of recurrence for all women; however, not every woman will need them. Boost treatments may use external beam therapy, or the radiation may be delivered internally with brachytherapy.

External Boost Treatments

The external boost treatments are similar to the standard external beam treatments; however, the area being treated will be smaller. These boost treatments are usually given daily for one week.

Internal Boost Treatments

The internal boost treatments with brachytherapy may be an option for a woman who has had a lumpectomy. The radiation is delivered to the tumor site from inside the breast. Brachytherapy begins with the surgical insertion of multiple tiny catheters into the area from which the tumor was surgically removed. Then, during a treatment, a radioactive seed is delivered into each catheter.

The brachytherapy may be given at a "high-dose rate" or a "low-dose rate." The difference between the two doses relates to the time it takes to complete the treatments. The high-dose-rate brachytherapy is given on an outpatient basis, twice a day for two to five days; each treatment usually lasts a few minutes. The low-dose brachytherapy is given continuously over a two-day period on an inpatient basis.

After the treatment is completed, the tiny catheters are removed. If you must travel to a radiation facility for treatment, brachytherapy reduces the number of days you will need to travel.

Accelerated Partial Breast Irradiation

A newer form of treatment, *accelerated partial breast irradiation (APBI),* is becoming an increasingly popular form of radiation treatment for women who have had lumpectomies. APBI can be delivered with external beam radiation or with brachytherapy. It delivers radiation only to the lumpectomy site rather than the whole breast. As a result, the treatment minimizes radiation exposure to healthy tissue, and the treatment takes only about five days rather than several weeks. It can also be delivered prior to chemotherapy. Most women report few side effects.

Who is a candidate for partial breast irradiation? Generally, good candidates are women with smaller tumors who have clear surgical margins, have only one site of cancer, and have minimal lymph node involvement.

Is APBI effective? Yes it is, according to a 2009 study done at the William Beaumont Hospital in Michigan. This study, which followed up with women ten years after their treatments, showed the same low rate of recurrence (5 percent) among women who received whole breast radiation and those who received partial breast radiation.

Radiation Therapy Side Effects

Because radiation is a localized treatment, it typically has only localized side effects. The majority of women go through radiation treatment with few or minimal side effects. The potential temporary side effects of radiation include:

- swelling of the area
- skin redness, resembling a sunburn
- discomfort in the treated area (This is not a sign of cancer recurring.)
- fatigue

There is the potential for long-term side effects after radiation therapy. These may include:

- reduced skin elasticity
- a breast that is firmer than normal
- puffiness or change in the size of the treated breast
- change in sensitivity to touch or pressure

- slight darkening or thickening of the skin
- chronic twinges or slight aching in the breast
- arm lymphedema (if lymph nodes received radiation)

Other complications are not likely, but are possible. Tenderness of the chest wall and rib fracture are possible, but are rare. *Radiation pneumonitis* is a lung reaction that may occur during treatment or weeks to months after treatment; it causes fever, coughing, and shortness of breath. It usually does not require treatment and goes away in a few weeks. It is also possible for radiation therapy to damage the heart; however, modern treatments strive to avoid this. Women who smoke or who have preexisting heart disease may be more at risk for a heart ailment. Finally, women under age forty-five have a slight risk (1 in 1,000) for developing cancer five to twenty years later; such cancer may develop in the skin, muscle, bone, or lung.

Radiation therapy for breast cancer will not affect your fertility, menstrual periods, or reproductive system. Some women can breastfeed with the untreated breast and sometimes with the treated breast.

Tips for Self-Care

Take especially good care of yourself during the time you're undergoing radiation treatments. These self-care basics can ease your side effects and keep you more comfortable:

- Get plenty of rest.
- Use lukewarm water and fragrance-free soap to cleanse the treated area. Do not scrub.
- Wear loose, comfortable clothing during the weeks of treatment. If possible, don't wear a bra.
- Don't use powders on the treated area before a treatment.

- Ask your radiation oncologist to recommend a skin cream to use on treated skin after treatments.
- Shield the treated area from sunlight. Some physicians recommend wearing protective clothing or using sunscreen for up to a year following radiation treatment.
- Don't try to scrub or rub off the ink marks that may have been applied at the time of your simulation or at your daily treatments. The marks will fade in time. Tattoos, however, don't fade but they can be removed professionally afterward with a laser.

These measures may help keep you comfortable, lift your spirits, manage your side effects, and help you feel more in control during this time of healing.

7

CHEMOTHERAPY, HORMONE THERAPY, AND TARGETED THERAPY

After breast cancer surgery, it's possible for some cancer cells to still remain in the body. Therefore, *systemic therapy* is recommended in some cases. Systemic therapy drugs travel through the bloodstream (throughout the body's system) to fight cancer.

One of the systemic treatments you may be most familiar with is *chemotherapy,* which works to destroy undetected cancer cells that may have spread to areas beyond the location of the original tumor. In addition to discussing chemotherapy for breast cancer, this chapter will also examine *hormone-blocking therapy* and *targeted therapy.*

Your Medical Oncologist

Chemotherapy is administered by a medical oncologist, a physician who specializes in systemic cancer treatments. Your surgeon will refer you to a well-qualified medical oncologist in your area. This physician should be board-certified in medical oncology. To be board-certified, a doctor must have the prescribed training and pass rigorous examinations. This specialist should be someone who inspires your confidence, listens carefully to your questions and concerns, and puts you at ease. You may find it helpful to arrive at each appointment with a list of your questions.

It is important for your doctor to know what medications you are taking, including prescription drugs, vitamins, herbs, and over-the-counter drugs such as aspirin, ibuprofen, sleep aids, and cold medicines.

Chemotherapy

The term *chemotherapy* refers to a group of drugs. Chemotherapy drugs have different modes of action against cancer cells, so doctors prescribe them in combinations that maximize their benefits. Combining drugs achieves higher remission rates and better disease-free survival rates.

After surgery and chemotherapy, I also had radiation. I got great support from family and friends. I kept telling myself I would beat this disease.

—Shirley, 58

The decision to use chemotherapy depends on such factors as the type of tumor, how aggressive it is, and a patient's age and overall health. Chemotherapy is often recommended when cancer has spread from the breast to the underarm lymph nodes and is routinely recommended when a tumor has aggressive characteristics, whether or not the lymph nodes are cancerous. With very small (about two inches) aggressive tumors with no evidence of cancer in the nodes, chemotherapy is prescribed only on a case-by-case basis; it may not be needed, especially if the cancer diagnosis was made early.

Chemotherapy Treatments

There are chemotherapy drugs that you can take at home in pill, capsule, or liquid form. More often, however, chemotherapy drugs are injected or infused (slowly dripped); occasionally, the chemotherapy is injected into a muscle, under the skin, or into the cancer itself. Only a medical professional, trained and experienced in the use

Chemotherapy Treatment

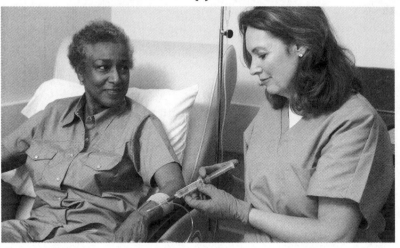

Most chemotherapy treatments are delivered intravenously. Treatments are usually given after surgery, but are sometimes given to shrink a tumor prior to surgery.

of chemotherapy, can administer drugs in this way, so each treatment requires a visit to the oncologist's office.

When chemotherapy is infused, it is usually given through a vein with an intravenous (IV) line or through a small port that leads into a vein. The port, about the size of a quarter, is made of plastic or metal, and is surgically implanted just under the skin. A soft tube, called a *catheter,* runs from the port to a large vein; the port remains in place until all chemotherapy treatments are finished.

The port has several advantages. It's usually more convenient for patients since it eliminates the need for repeated needle "sticks." A port is also useful for the delivery of certain medications or when an infusion over several days is needed. It's also useful when conditions such as swelling or obesity make it difficult for medical professionals to find a vein. Also, some chemotherapy drugs can be damaging to veins and soft tissue, so a port is essential when these drugs are prescribed.

If you receive chemotherapy, the dose will be customized especially for you. The goal is to kill as many

Five Decades of Chemotherapy

Chemotherapy has been used to treat breast cancer since the late 1960s. However, it was during the 1970s that its curative powers became known. During this time, chemotherapy was determined to be an effective treatment for women whose breast cancers had spread to nearby lymph nodes. The medical community also learned chemotherapy dramatically decreased a woman's rate of breast cancer recurrence. The increase in the survival rate was striking, and by the 1990s, chemotherapy was recommended for women with stages I through III breast cancer.

cancer cells as possible without putting you at undue risk. There is a small range of acceptable dosages, but within that range, there is room for differences of opinion. Some oncologists prefer to give the highest acceptable dosages; others prefer to give lower dosages more often. As a consequence, your treatments might be weekly, every other week, or even monthly. The nature of each drug and drug combination also determines how often it is given.

Timing of Chemotherapy Cycles

The earlier chemotherapy is given after surgery, the better; there will be fewer cancer cells to attack and the likelihood of success is enhanced. A common chemotherapy regimen begins two to four weeks after surgery and continues for three months to six months.

There is a reason why chemotherapy is given in cycles. This approach kills more cancer cells. The first cycle of treatment will kill many cells that are in the process of dividing; it will miss cells that are at rest, but will kill some of these in the next cycle. These cycles of treatment continue with the intent of destroying as many remaining cancer cells as possible. The number and duration of cycles depend on the drugs being used, their dosages, and the stage of the cancer.

Most chemotherapy is given after surgery; however, in some cases, it is better to give the chemotherapy prior to surgery. This approach is called *neoadjuvant chemotherapy.* The intent of this therapy is to shrink a tumor prior to surgical removal. This form of chemotherapy is always recommended for inflammatory breast cancer and other forms of aggressive breast cancers. Chemotherapy prior to surgery may also be recommended to shrink a tumor if a woman is interested in having a lumpectomy rather than having a breast removed.

Breast cancer is like speed bumps in the road. You have rough days or rough procedures, but it gets better. You get over them.
—*Kristine, 51*

Side Effects of Chemotherapy

Despite the advances in chemotherapy over the years, you'll probably feel a little nervous at first about side effects. It might help to remember that these side effects are only temporary. Side effects vary widely among patients and among various drugs. Not everyone will have problems with nausea and hair loss. You might be on a different chemotherapy regimen and schedule. You might react differently to the drugs being used, and you might be given different medications to control your side effects.

Fatigue

Fatigue is common during chemotherapy treatments and may have many causes. It may be caused by a low count in red blood cells; these cells carry the oxygen that gives the body fuel for energy, so a reduction in red blood cells causes fatigue and sometimes shortness of breath and light-headedness. Women who experience fatigue during the course of their chemotherapy treatments say the second or third day after treatment is often the most difficult, but the fatigue often lessens in subsequent days.

A flexible schedule helps. If you find yourself tired late in the day, try making time for a nap before dinner. Fatigue may increase as the months of chemotherapy progress, and it may persist for a year or two after treatment ends.

In cases where fatigue is caused by low red blood counts, your oncologist may prescribe drugs that stimulate production of red or white blood cells.

Infections

White blood cells fight infection, and when chemotherapy causes a reduction of white blood cells, the risk of infection increases. Signs of infection, such as fever, chills, redness of skin, pain, or swelling, should be promptly reported to your medical oncologist.

If your white blood cell count gets dangerously low, your doctor might briefly postpone your chemotherapy treatment or lower your dosage. Alternatively, he or she might recommend an injection of a growth factor that causes bone marrow to produce and release more white blood cells, enabling you to remain on your normal chemotherapy dosage and schedule. Even so, you will be particularly vulnerable to infection during periods when your white blood cell counts are low.

Bruising or Bleeding

Chemotherapy can cause a drop in one's level of blood platelets—cells that aid in blood clotting. When these platelet levels drop, you may have nosebleeds or bleeding gums. Or, you may bruise easily or bleed longer if you cut or nick your skin. If any of these symptoms occurs, notify your doctor right away.

Changes in Weight

Weight loss. Losing weight sometimes occurs as a side effect of chemotherapy. Lack of appetite may occur as a result of poor appetite or nausea. Quick weight loss of five pounds in a week may be a sign of dehydration and should be reported to your doctor immediately. It is recommended that you keep track of your weight, weighing each morning before eating or drinking.

Weight gain. You may be surprised to learn that nearly half the women undergoing chemotherapy gain weight. Factors that may cause an increase in weight: reduction in exercise, the body holding on to excess fluids, food cravings, and slowing of metabolism—the rate at which the body uses energy. Other drugs, such as steroids for side effects, can cause weight gain. Also, hormone therapy that decreases levels of the hormones estrogen and progesterone can cause weight gain.

I had two rounds of chemotherapy and radiation. But every day puts you in a better place. The greatest lesson I learned was that hard times don't last. You will feel better. Things will get better.

—Ann, 53

Nausea

Nausea has not been completely eliminated as a side effect of chemotherapy. However, fewer and fewer patients experience nausea during chemotherapy, but those who do can usually manage it well with over-the-counter medicines or prescription drugs. Many anti-nausea drugs are now available. Your medical oncologist will prescribe them.

Another tip for avoiding nausea: eat slowly and eat small amounts of food at a time. Dry foods such as toast or crackers may help relieve nausea. Eating heavily the day of treatment and several days afterward is not advised.

For those patients who do experience nausea, their physicians may also recommend hydration (fluids and medications) through an IV. Many oncologists have services available seven days a week. Check with your oncologist about such services.

Hair Loss

Why do some chemotherapy drugs cause hair loss? The answer is simple: cancer cells are rapidly dividing cells, and chemotherapy is designed to kill rapidly dividing cells. Hair cells are also rapidly dividing cells, so they, too, are affected by chemotherapy. This explains why hair often falls out during chemotherapy.

Losing hair is one of the side effects that women find especially emotionally painful. However, the hair not only grows back, but it's not uncommon for the new hair to be thicker, curlier, or even a slightly different color. In some women, the hair only gets thinner rather than falls out completely. Hair loss or thinning can start a few days after chemotherapy begins, but two or three weeks later is more usual.

If you do lose your hair—including eyebrows, lashes, and body hair—it will probably grow back within three to five months after you complete chemotherapy. Regrowth sometimes starts even before chemotherapy has ended. However, incomplete hair regrowth has been reported occasionally. Before starting chemotherapy, discuss this with your oncologist.

Before your treatment begins, you might want to buy an attractive hairpiece that matches your hair color and is cut and styled the way you like it. Stock up on hats, scarves, and turbans if you find wigs too uncomfortable. Being prepared will help you manage hair loss if it does occur.

A program called "Look Good...Feel Better" (www.lookgoodfeelbetter.org) puts cancer patients in touch with cosmetologists who provide free advice on makeup and wigs. For more information, *see* the American Cancer Society listing in the Resources section at the back of this book.

Another approach, cooling of the scalp with a cooling cap, will reduce hair loss caused by some chemotherapy drugs but not all. A cooling cap tightens blood vessels in the scalp; this action may reduce the effects of chemotherapy on hair follicles and prevent or reduce hair loss. If you are concerned about hair loss, discuss this with your oncologist.

I didn't want to go through chemo; I didn't want to lose my hair, but I did. Later, at stop signs, I used to whip off my wig on the hot drives home from work and enjoy the astonishment on the faces of other drivers.

—*Suzanne, 58*

Memory Loss

Some women having chemotherapy report a condition called "chemo brain" or "brain fog" that may start during treatment or after. This "fog" is refers to problems with memory, attention, and thinking. Some women say they are forgetful or "fuzzy-headed" and find it harder to concentrate. The condition is almost always mild and short-lived; however, for some women, the condition can last for years.

Study results haven't been unanimous on the cause of this memory loss. Some researchers believe that the problem is a direct result of some chemotherapy drugs as well as other cancer treatments. Others claim that the memory problems have more to do with hormonal changes, sleep disruption, and the emotional trauma of being diagnosed with and treated for breast cancer.

Menopausal Symptoms

Some women stop menstruating during chemotherapy and also may experience the night sweats and hot flashes common in menopause. Other menopausal symptoms include vaginal dryness, fatigue, depression, insomnia, and weight gain.

Younger women usually begin menstruating again after chemotherapy, but women older than forty may not. For those who do resume menstruating, fertility is not thought to be affected; it is still possible to conceive and bear children. Remember, temporary cessation of menses during chemotherapy does not necessarily mean you are infertile. So use appropriate non-hormonal birth control measures to prevent pregnancy because chemotherapy drugs can cause birth defects.

Joint Pain

After chemotherapy, about 5 percent of patients notice short-term or lasting joint pain. Most physicians recommend over-the-counter anti-inflammatory drugs such as ibuprofen. Some doctors say their patients report success in relieving joint pain with the over-the-counter supplements chondroitin and glucosamine or fish oil, which are available at most pharmacies and health food stores. Dietary changes may also be beneficial—eating low-carb foods along with fruits and vegetables. Studies have also proven that exercise reduces joint pain, so a regular exercise program is important.

Other Side Effects of Chemotherapy

Other side effects from chemotherapy can include mouth sores and taste changes, poor appetite, diarrhea or constipation, tingling or numbness in the hands or feet, irritated skin, fluid retention, and brittle nails. Discuss these side effects with your doctor, especially if they are persistent or get worse.

Side effects from chemotherapy aren't insignificant, but they need not put your life on hold. Chemotherapy has improved to the point where many working women continue working during the course of their treatments. And if you just don't feel up to staying on the job, or you'd rather work part-time on a flexible schedule, discuss your options with your employer.

Hormone-Blocking Therapy

Hormone-blocking therapy works much differently than chemotherapy. Rather than destroying cancer cells, hormone-blocking drugs keep cancer cells from reproducing. Breast cancers that are "fed" by estrogen is called *estrogen positive breast cancer;* if the cancer is fed by the hormone progesterone, it is referred to as *progesterone positive*. Hormone-blocking drugs can literally starve cancers of these hormones, which the cancer needs to survive. The therapy does this in one of two ways—by interfering with the body's production of estrogen, by attaching to the hormone receptors of cancer cells or by altering the hormone receptor on the cancer cell itself. Either way, the cancer cell dies without hormones to feed it.

I thought if there's a chance chemotherapy will kill any cancer left in my body, the six-month inconvenience was worth it.
—*Dianna, 44*

Hormone-blocking therapy is prescribed when blood tests show that hormone receptors are present, regardless of tumor size or lymph node involvement. One of the advantages of hormone-blocking therapy is that the drugs act against cancer cells without significant effects on normal cells, making these drugs easier to tolerate than chemotherapy drugs.

Hormone-blocking therapy given after surgery improves a woman's prognosis by reducing the possibility of the same cancer recurring and also reducing the probability that a new cancer will develop. With regular follow-up, the benefits of hormone-blocking therapy are likely to continue at least fifteen years after the five- to ten-year treatment period. In selected cases, hormone therapy can also be used before surgery to shrink tumors.

Side Effects of Hormone-Blocking Drugs

Your doctor will give you a list of possible side effects of hormone-blocking drugs. Possible side effects include

> ## Immunotherapy for Breast Cancer
> In past years, immunotherapy treatments have not been available to treat breast cancer; however, that changed in early 2019, when, for the first time, the FDA approved an immunotherapy drug that may be used for treating breast cancer.
>
> Immunotherapy drugs may be given to stimulate your own immune system to fight cancer. Or, you may be given drugs, called *immune system proteins,* that help the body fight cancer. These treatments are often referred to as *biologic therapy* or *biotherapy.*

vaginal dryness, fatigue, nausea, depression, hot flashes, weight gain, insomnia, and memory loss.

Some hormone-blocking drugs have been linked to a slightly higher risk of uterine cancer. Also, you should not take certain hormone-blocking drugs if you have a history of blood clots. Some classes of drugs may cause dry eyes and contribute to the development of cataracts; however, this is an extremely rare side effect with today's lower doses. Some drugs can also cause deposits in the retina at the back of the eye. You should have regular eye exams while you are on hormone-blocking drugs.

Targeted Therapy

Another form of systemic treatment, *targeted therapy,* involves using drugs to defend against cancer by attaching to specific molecules within or on the surface of cancer cells. As the name implies, targeted cancer therapies target specific characteristics of cancer cells, such as a protein that enables cancer cells to grow. Because targeted therapies attack cancer cells only, they are less likely than chemotherapy to harm normal, healthy cells.

As the medical community has learned more about the gene changes in cells that cause cancer, they have been able to develop drugs that target these changes. Some targeted-therapy drugs represent truly astonishing accomplishments in genetic engineering.

Several targeted therapy drugs work to destroy breast cancers that are referred to as "HER2 positive." You may recall from chapter 2, HER2 is a protein that appears in or on the surface of cancer cells; this protein causes cancer to grow and spread. Targeted therapy drugs work on the surface of cancer cells by blocking the chemical signals that can stimulate cancer growth.

Targeted therapy drugs may be given alone or with chemotherapy. These drugs are usually given intravenously in a hospital or an infusion center. Receiving an infusion will usually take from thirty to ninety minutes, depending on your dosage, the frequency of your infusions, and how well you tolerate the infusions.

Chemotherapy was relatively easy for me, and my family was considerate of my lack of energy. I bought a wig the same color as my hair and, for the most part, continued on with my life.
—*Carolyn, 65*

Side Effects of Targeted Therapy

Side effects are typically mild because healthy cells aren't damaged; however, side effects may include:

- skin problems and diarrhea (rash, dry skin, nail changes, change in hair color)
- problems with blood clotting and wound healing
- high blood pressure
- gastrointestinal perforation (a rare side effect of some targeted therapies)

In rare cases, a targeted therapy drug may cause heart failure. Oncologists guard against this by testing cardiac muscle function every twelve weeks; any changes in cardiac function are almost always reversible. And, a drug can be stopped until a patient gains full heart function with the help of heart-strengthening medications.

Immunotherapy is used most often in triple negative breast cancer. Studies are currently exploring the use of immunotherapy in other types of breast cancer.

Is Systemic Therapy Right for You?

The same types of breast cancers are often found in both younger, premenopausal women and older, postmenopausal women. However, as a general rule, younger women are more likely to have more aggressive breast cancers. As a result, younger women are more likely than older women to require chemotherapy when diagnosed with breast cancer. However, the actual treatment recommendation depends on the characteristics of the breast cancer as well as the overall health and age of the woman.

Research Continues

Scientists are pursuing targeted and immune therapies using many different mechanisms to combat cancer. Some work by replacing missing or defective genes with "good" copies of the gene, sometimes using viruses to transport the drugs. Other experimental targeted therapies use stem cells to deliver anticancer agents directly into tumor metastases. Vaccines are also being developed to find and destroy cancer-promoting proteins.

Along with new drugs, refinements in genetic and molecular profiling of breast cancer make it possible to tailor treatment for the type of breast cancer a woman has. If you are seeking treatment, it is most helpful to find a medical oncologist who is aware of the latest news in cancer research so you can be assured of receiving the most current therapy.

Treatments that were unimaginable twenty years ago are saving lives today. The basic science research that has been ongoing over the past two decades is now becoming clinically useful, with many new drugs approved for breast cancer over the past few years.

8

LOCAL RECURRENCE OF BREAST CANCER

If your breast cancer has responded well to treatment, you have every reason to celebrate—treatments have worked, you have survived, and you can move on with your life. However, if you are like most survivors, somewhere in the back of your mind you fear that the cancer will recur or that a new cancer will develop. *Local recurrence* is the return of cancer to the breast or chest wall on the side that the cancer first appeared. A *regional recurrence* refers to cancer appearing in the nearby armpit or collarbone area.

Some women first confront these kinds of fears when the initial shock of diagnosis wears off and surgery is over. Others don't begin worrying until they have finished radiation therapy or adjuvant therapy. When you stop making frequent visits to familiar doctors and nurses, you may feel strangely vulnerable. For example, you may feel a wave of anxiety with every small headache or bodily pain, certain that the cancer is back.

Fortunately, the anxieties subside with time. Most women begin relaxing a little after each checkup until two years, and then five, have finally passed. If breast cancer recurs, it is most likely to recur within the first five years. After the ten-year mark, a woman's risk of recurrence is greatly reduced.

Risk of Recurrence

Keep in mind that 70 to 90 percent of the women diagnosed with early-stage breast cancer never have a recurrence after treatment. Well over half of the women who experience a recurrence live ten years or more after treatment for the recurrence. Again, early detection is key: The sooner a new tumor is discovered, the better the chances for recovery. There's a great deal you can do to keep your body strong and less vulnerable to recurrence.

Chapter 1 discussed the general risks linked to primary breast cancer—the various environmental, hereditary, and behavioral factors thought to play a role in the development of this disease. To understand your risk of recurrence, consider these factors as well as the ones associated with your type of breast cancer.

The same cancer characteristics that were used to guide your initial treatments will also help to estimate your risk of recurrence. These characteristics include:

- Tumor size
- Lymph node involvement
- Presence or absence of hormone receptors
- Rate of cancer-cell division (Poorly differentiated cells divide rapidly; well-differentiated cells divide less rapidly.)
- Presence of micrometastases (small groups of breast cancer cells)
- *HER2/neu overexpression:* HER2/neu is a protein that can promote the growth of breast cancer cells. An increased production of the protein is known as *overexpression.*
- *BRCA1* or *BRCA2 gene mutation:* Everyone has BRCA1 and BRCA2 genes. Some people have an inherited mutation in one or both of these genes that increases the risk of breast cancer. The mutation can be inherited from either parent.

- *p53 tumor markers:* p53 is a gene that, when damaged, may be associated with a high risk of breast cancer. A marker is a substance in the blood or tissue that may indicate the presence of cancer.
- *Ki-67:* This protein's growth rate in cancer cells can be measured to help determine how fast a tumor is growing.

Symptoms of Local Recurrence

One of the best strategies for long-term survival is to pay close attention to your body. Use the information in this book and other sources so that you understand the signs and symptoms of breast cancer. Become familiar with the warning signs of breast cancer recurrence. The better you understand the actual warning signs, the more relaxed you'll probably be about unrelated symptoms. The follow are symptoms of a local recurrence:

- A new lump in the breast
- Firmness in a new part of the breast
- Swelling or redness of skin around the breast area
- Changes to the nipple
- Presence of bumps on or under the skin of the chest
- Thickening on or near a mastectomy scar
- Pulling of skin or swelling at the site of a lumpectomy

Ask your doctor about your specific risk of recurrence. Cancer, by definition, is unpredictable, so it's difficult to be certain how a cancer will behave.

Risk of a New Cancer

It is only fair to think that if you have had breast cancer once, you should not have to worry about it twice. But cancer is never fair, and sometimes a new primary cancer does develop; it may show up in a breast

---

Types of Recurring Breast Cancer

Local recurrence: the return of cancer to the breast or chest wall.

Regional recurrence: the return of cancer in the lymph nodes in the armpit or collarbone near the area where the cancer was originally detected.

Distant recurrence: cancer has spread beyond the breast and nearby lymph nodes to a distant part of the body. Also called *metastatic breast cancer. See* chapter 9.

---

treated with lumpectomy, in an untreated breast, or, less commonly, in a small amount of breast tissue left behind after mastectomy. Fortunately, the risk of a second breast cancer remains small. However, if you have had a very aggressive cancer, you may be more likely to develop a recurrence of breast cancer.

Some women have an inherited tendency to develop a series of primary cancers. Those who have this unusual condition might recover from breast cancer only to face other cancers in other parts of the body. For more information, talk with your oncologist or contact the Hereditary Cancer Center (*see* the Resources section at the back of this book).

Follow-Up Care

Physicians today have several strategies for reducing your risk of further cancer, and new strategies are being studied all the time. Your follow-up care will be more frequent and comprehensive during the first year or so after your surgery. Depending on the treatment you received, you'll visit your cancer surgeon, radiation oncologist, medical oncologist, and plastic surgeon (if you have had reconstruction).

Your primary physician, the one who has coordinated your care throughout your treatment, will probably be involved in your follow-up care as well. He or she should be in touch with all the members of your medical team throughout the follow-up period, and you'll probably

Preventing Cancer Recurrence
- Engage in three or more hours of moderate exercise each week.
- Eat a balanced, healthful diet.
- Control weight.
- Avoid alcohol.
- Control blood sugar, if diabetic.

see your primary care doctor every six months for a complete physical examination. Any member of your team of physicians may order diagnostic tests as part of your follow-up care.

Blood Tests

After you have had *systemic treatment* (chemotherapy, targeted therapy, or hormonal therapy), you'll probably have monthly blood tests. Your doctor will use blood tests to look for tumor markers, high amounts of substances, such as certain proteins, that might indicate when a tumor is present. The tests are not sensitive enough to find a recurrence at its earliest stages because a tumor must be large enough to release detectable amounts of the marker substances.

Blood test results sometimes include false negatives; this means test results may look normal when, in fact, cancer cells may be present. Thus, the most appropriate use of these tests is in following a known recurrence to gauge its response to therapy.

Other blood tests look for elevated levels of enzymes that sometimes indicate the presence of cancer in the liver or bone. If blood test results suggest a problem with the liver, you may have a PET/CT scan to investigate further. If tests show that bone cancer could be present, or if you experience bone pain, your doctor may order a bone scan.

Scans

The first step in a *bone scan* is injection of a radioactive liquid into the bloodstream. After a few hours, the radioactive particles are absorbed by the bones, where they concentrate in areas of increased blood circulation that could indicate cancer. Such areas, called "hot spots," are detected by a machine that scans your body from above while you are lying on a table. Hot spots can appear for many reasons—injury, arthritis, or other problems besides cancer cells—and the machine cannot distinguish the cause. Therefore, if a bone scan shows an area of increased blood circulation, it may require follow-up with an X-ray, PET/CT scan, or MRI, which can show more clearly what is going on at that site.

PET and CT scan. This scan combines the PET scan with a CT scan, each part of the test providing different information. The PET scan shows areas of increased metabolic activity while the CT scan shows physical details. Both scans are done at the same time, and the process takes a little under two hours.

Computerized tomography (CT) uses radiation to display cross sections of the body, which can reveal cancers deep within the body or brain. During the scan, you'll need to lie very still while the CT machine takes X-ray pictures from many different angles. A computer assembles these slices of images into a detailed picture of the scanned area. A CT scan takes only a few minutes to complete.

Magnetic resonance imaging (MRI). An MRI uses a magnetic field instead of X-rays to take many pictures from a variety of angles. The MRI can find soft-tissue abnormalities that other tests may overlook.

Chest X-Rays

Breast cancer survivors may be advised to have a chest X-ray if they experience shortness of breath or a persistent cough. A chest X-ray may determine whether breast cancer has spread to the lungs. Metastasis in the lungs does not usually cause pain, but it can cause a stubborn cough or shortness of breath.

I always wonder if the cancer will return. I don't always talk about it, but the scare is there at times. One day at a time…that's how you live with cancer.

—*Liz, 42*

Breast Self-Examination and Mammography

Self-examination and mammograms remain critical after cancer treatment. If you have had a lumpectomy, you should examine both breasts and the entire breast area, as outlined in chapter 2. If you have had a mastectomy, you should examine your untreated breast, the surgical site, and the surrounding area, paying attention to your incision and chest wall for thickness, lumps, or rigidity. Report any suspicious changes to your doctor immediately.

Most experts recommend a mammogram about six months after treatment. If you have had a lumpectomy, a mammogram of the surgically treated breast will serve as a new reference point to which your doctor will compare future mammograms. The other breast will look about the same on the new image as on earlier ones. If you have had a mastectomy, a physical examination of your incision, armpit, breast area, and the area above your collarbone will be sufficient, but you should have routine mammograms done on your opposite breast. Most physicians recommend mammograms every six months for the first year and then annually after that.

Hormone-Blocking Therapy

If your original tumor tested positive for hormone receptors, you probably began a five-to-ten-year course of hormone-blocking therapy, which kills cancer cells by keeping them from dividing. These hormone-blocking drugs have been shown to prevent primary breast cancer in some high-risk women, and they can also help keep cancer from recurring in women who have already had breast cancer. These drugs also shrink existing tumors and are used to prevent breast cancer metastases. Like all anticancer drugs, they have risks and side effects as well as benefits. Ask your doctor to discuss these with you.

I chose a double mastectomy because I didn't want to have to worry about recurrence. I am glad I made the decision.

—Billie, 48

Treatment for Local Recurrence

Cancer that reappears after lumpectomy, at the site of the original tumor, is one form of local recurrence. Radiation isn't usually an option for treating the cancer, since you probably will have had radiation after your lumpectomy; repeated radiation would cause too much tissue damage. Your doctor will probably want to perform a mastectomy as the best way of removing all the cancer. However, if radiation was not used to treat your initial cancer, an option may be a second lumpectomy followed by radiation.

Local recurrence after mastectomy can appear in the surgical scar, in the skin or fat where the breast was, in the muscle or bone of the chest wall, or in a remnant of breast tissue left behind after the surgery. Surgery is the first line of treatment to remove the cancer and any affected tissue, muscle, or bone. If you didn't have radiation to the site after your mastectomy, radiation can now be used on the entire chest wall to eradicate any microscopic traces of the cancer.

Most cases of local recurrence are treated locally, with surgery and in some cases radiation. If the original tumor tested positive for hormone receptors, hormone blocking therapy, along with other drugs, will likely be recommended. But if there is evidence of metastatic disease, a tissue biopsy will be tested for hormone receptors. Treatment may call for hormone-blocking therapy, chemotherapy, a combination of both, or immunotherapy.

Self-Care

Whether your cancer recurs or you worry that it will, there are many things you can do to boost your confidence, protect your well-being, and feel in control over important aspects of your life. Many breast cancer survivors suggest living one day at a time, paying attention to the things that matter most—eating well, exercising, meditating, pursuing a spiritual search, finding creative expression, and nurturing the relationships that sustain you.

Do things that fuel your energy and give you the greatest satisfaction. Try to reestablish routines and challenges that were interrupted by your illness. Add new ones, ways of reaching out and enriching your life.

As mentioned previously, a support group can offer priceless help and new friendships. Consider working with organizations that promote breast cancer awareness and research. You might work with survivors like yourself or with women just recently diagnosed, who need to see what you represent—life going on after cancer.

Activism has been responsible for many strides against breast cancer in recent years. You could make a difference by battling this disease on a new front, even in small ways. There is always something you can do. Your life remains your own.

9

METASTATIC
BREAST CANCER

If your medical oncologist tells you that you have *metastatic breast cancer,* it means your breast cancer has spread beyond the breast and nearby lymph nodes to a distant part of your body.

Metastatic breast cancer is not usually cured, but it can be controlled. By learning the makeup of cancer cells—their characteristics—your oncologist can offer smarter, personalized treatment to keep any cancer cells in check for months, if not years. Because of today's drug therapies, people with metastatic breast cancer are living longer, satisfying, quality lives with progression-free disease.

Let's take a closer look at what else you should know about metastatic breast cancer to navigate your diagnosis and disease.

Understanding the Basics

Metastatic breast cancer, or *advanced breast cancer,* occurs when microscopic cancerous cells break away from a primary or original tumor, invading nearby healthy tissue, then move through the blood or lymphatic systems to other organs. New metastases or tumors grow in those locations. Metastasis to the bone is common, but may also develop in the lungs, liver, or brain.

About 70 percent of metastatic breast cancers involve the spread of cancer to bones. Bone metastasis can occur in any bone but more commonly occurs in the spine, pelvis, and thigh. Wherever the cancer has spread, however, it is still considered and treated as breast cancer rather than as a primary cancer in the location to which it has spread. For example, if breast cancer should appear in the ribs or spine, it isn't bone cancer. It's metastatic breast cancer.

Rare, But Still a Risk

Statistics suggest that metastatic breast cancer is relatively rare, especially as an initial diagnosis. Only about 5 percent of new breast cancer cases have already spread beyond the breast when first diagnosed as *stage IV* cancer. The incidence rises over time, however. Between 10 to 15 percent of patients eventually develop a recurrence of their disease, sometimes years after receiving a cancer-free stage I, II, or III prognosis.

Despite those statistics, the individual risk of cancer returning and spreading varies among women, depending on a variety of factors including an original tumor's profile, biology, and stage. Individuals diagnosed initially with aggressive forms of breast cancer have a high risk of their cancer recurring within the first few years.

Other women may not experience metastatic disease for many years because it's slow-growing. A recurrence may be a decade down the road. If you're estrogen-positive, for instance, you may respond favorably to hormone treatment, but still have dormant diseased cells. Estrogen-positive means cancer cells are "fed" by the hormones estrogen and progesterone. If your breast cancer has a significant number of receptors for either of these hormones, it's considered *hormone-receptor positive.*

Even with today's sophisticated diagnostic techniques, physicians don't have a singular test to tell you if you're destined to develop metastatic breast cancer or which organ might be involved. However, doctors have some indicators. For example, between 10 and 15 percent of stage IV cancer patients experience metastatic brain tumors, with most occurring after the cancer has migrated to other parts of the body. Still, no one can predict exactly where and when metastatic disease will occur, much less who will be diagnosed with it.

You have to be an advocate for your own health.
If you notice a change in your breast or a change in how you are feeling, get checked. We'd much rather have a false alarm than miss something important.
—*Stephen, medical oncologist*

Symptoms of Metastatic Breast Cancer

Symptoms of metastatic breast cancer vary, depending on where and how far your cancer has spread and what type of tissue is now involved. You may experience a variety of general signs—fatigue, poor appetite, and weight loss—that your medical oncologist will want to investigate. But he or she will focus primarily on those symptoms that indicate the location of the cancer in the body.

Don't panic if you have these symptoms. Many times these symptoms do not mean cancer; but do see your physician.

Bone Pain

Sudden or progressive severe pain plus swelling at a specific spot may indicate that your bones are affected. Since a bone metastasis puts you at higher risk for fractures, the discomfort could indicate a fracture. Numbness and weakness or even difficulty with urination or bowel movements may suggest that the fracture involves the vertebrae or bones in the spinal cord, causing it to pinch nerves that control those functions.

Coughing, Chest Pain

If breast cancer has spread to the lungs, you may not have any immediate symptoms; sometimes cancer in a lung is discovered during a routine follow-up chest X-ray or other imaging test. If you have symptoms, however, they'll likely be similar to persistent, upper respiratory infections: coughing, chest pain, shortness of breath, or difficulty breathing.

Jaundice

Cancer that is affecting your liver may cause jaundice, which is a yellow tinge to your skin and the whites of your eyes. Discoloration can be accompanied by an itchy rash and swollen hands or feet. Tests may also reveal abnormally high liver enzymes, which indicate that the organ is being damaged.

Headaches, Memory Problems

Breast cancer that's spread to part of your nervous system, brain, or spinal cord can cause any number of symptoms: persistently bad or worsening headaches, memory problems, and mood or personality changes, plus slurred speech, visual issues, and dizziness. You may also experience seizures or signs of a stroke, such as a sudden one-sided weakness and numbness.

If you notice any new symptom, make sure to contact your physician without delay. Don't just assume that it's your arthritis kicking up or the flu. Sometimes it's hard to distinguish between simple medical problems and more serious issues related to your cancer. But if you have intense pain that appears suddenly or other symptoms that linger for a week or two, call your physician. Your complaint may mean another health issue entirely, but if your cancer has metastasized, you want to address it immediately.

Getting a Diagnosis

Just as your cancer was initially diagnosed with various tests, your medical oncologist will order various tests to determine the diagnosis of metastatic breast cancer. You've already read about the role of imaging, blood screens, and tissue biopsies in identifying a primary tumor, then using that information to personalize treatment. A similar process follows a diagnosis of metastatic disease. Your physician wants to know as much as possible about your cancer's unique characteristics in order to recommend the best therapy.

Imaging Tests

X-rays and ultrasounds plus CT, MRI, and PET scanning are important in getting "photos" of your brain, chest, abdomen, pelvis, spine, and long bones, areas to which cancer may have spread. Combining tests may be recommended to achieve the best picture possible. If your symptoms point to metastatic breast cancer in the bone, for instance, your oncologist will likely call for a CT whole-body scan with or without X-rays of specific skeletal structures. You may also undergo further PET and/or MRI testing. Likewise, if your liver is affected, expect scans such as ultrasound, MRI, CT, or PET. A chest CT or PET scan is usually ordered for the lung and an MRI for the brain or the spinal cord.

Blood Tests

Your medical oncologist will use various blood tests to find signs of metastatic disease. A comprehensive blood count and metabolic panel assesses your overall health and that of individual organs; blood tests are also used to examine your body's chemistry and the way it uses energy.

Also, testing for tumor markers can yield microscopic evidence that your cancer has spread. Tumor markers are substances, often proteins that are produced by cancer tissue or sometimes by the body as a result of cancer growth. Some of these substances are found in blood, urine, and tissue. These markers help detect and diagnose some types of cancer; they can also help in monitoring one's response to treatment.

Other chemicals released by various organs into your blood may reveal that new activities are occurring in the body. For example, high levels of calcium may indicate bone metastasis. The same is true with elevated hormone receptors and HER2. As explained earlier, HER2 is a protein that can play a role in the development of breast cancer. If your breast cancer tests show the presence of the HER2 protein, the breast cancer is said to be HER2 positive.

Tissue Biopsy

A tissue sample not only can confirm that your breast cancer has spread, but can also help your oncology team learn more about its cells. Even if you've been treated for an earlier cancer, your physician will want to biopsy or remove a small amount of tissue from your lymph nodes or a suspicious area for microscopic examination. Keep in mind that metastatic breast cancer is not always identical to an original breast cancer. In some women, the biology changes.

So, it's standard to test for any characteristics that not only help identify the type of cancer, but also indicate the best treatment choice. These characteristics include both hormone receptor and HER2 status. As mentioned previously, an abundance of estrogen and progesterone, along with the HER2 protein, can stimulate breast cancer cells to grow and spread. The same holds true in metastatic breast cancer. Knowing the cancer characteristics can help your physician determine which drugs will likely stop these new cancerous cells from reproducing.

Controlling Metastatic Breast Cancer

When breast cancer has spread to another part of the body, treatment must be as aggressive as possible, while keeping side effects tolerable. The same therapies are available for metastases as for a primary cancer—surgery, radiation (in areas not previously irradiated), and systemic therapies—though they may be used in different combinations or sequences than with a primary cancer.

When breast cancer has metastasized to the bone, lung, or liver, the first treatment is always systemic drugs—those that affect all parts of the body. That may include hormone therapy, targeted therapy, or chemotherapy or a combination of these drugs. Metastatic disease to the brain is usually treated with radiation and occasionally surgery.

Your medical oncologist won't likely know for several months whether your cancer is responding to treatment. But the general principle is that you stay on the regimen until your disease starts progressing or side effects are problematic. If that happens, your treatment may be followed by other medications as long as they are effective. For many women this approach leads to long-term progression-free disease.

Radiation may also be recommended for specific reasons such as alleviating localized pain or treating a target cancerous spot. However, radiation is used selectively. Physicians are concerned that if radiation is applied to too many areas of the body, it eventually destroys enough bone-marrow cells that you can't have chemotherapy in the future.

Surgery is not commonly used to treat metastatic breast cancer; however, in some cases, it may be recommended.

Tailoring Your Treatment Plan

In tailoring the best plan for you, your medical oncologist will take several variables into consideration, including your overall health and pre- or postmenopausal status. Whether your treatment involves combined medications or a single drug, your metastatic cancer's unique biology, especially its hormone-receptor and HER2 status, will be factors. If you have a BRCA gene mutation, you may also benefit from a class of drugs called *PARP inhibitors,* which are described later in this chapter.

Hormone Therapy

If your metastatic breast cancer is hormone-positive, or fueled by hormones, the treatment goal will be to slow the disease by interrupting hormones from influencing its cells. Your physician will prescribe hormone (endocrine therapy) medications that starve a tumor of the estrogen and progesterone it needs to survive and spread. Just to review, these therapies work in various ways. Drugs known as *SERMs (selective estrogen receptor modulators)* block estrogen from stimulating cell growth in tissues. Other drugs, such as *aromatase inhibitors,* halt estrogen production so that it can't feed cancer cells. Drugs known as *CDK inhibitors* (described in the next section) are often prescribed with hormone blockers and can nearby double the response time.

Still other drugs change the number of estrogen receptors on the surface of a cell, which stops cancerous cells from working. By depriving the cancer of functional hormones it needs, hormone therapy is generally successful in controlling metastatic breast cancer. Individuals often have long, progression-free survival, even a decade or more.

If your metastasized cancer is HER2-positive, your medical oncologist must consider the fact that metastatic breast cancer cells are producing too much of the protein HER2 and it's telling your tumor to keep growing. You'll likely undergo HER2-targeted therapy with drugs called *HER2 inhibitors* and *HER2 monoclonal antibodies.* These drugs either stall proteins within the cell from fueling HER2 growth or block the cells from receiving outside signals that do the same. Other medications combine man-made antibodies with chemotherapy. Because anti-HER2 therapy alone isn't always as effective in treating metastatic disease in earlier-stage breast cancer, the therapy is usually paired with other treatments.

Targeted Therapies

Your physician has several other drug options for treating metastatic disease, depending again on the cancer's cellular characteristics. As discussed earlier, targeted therapy disables cancerous cells by zeroing in on specific proteins and other molecules that determine how cells grow, survive, and spread. When combined with other medications such as hormone therapy, the drugs take out those mechanisms that are interfering with normal cellular growth.

CDK4/6 inhibitors. These drugs restore cell division control by switching off a protein called *cyclin-dependent kinase.* In healthy breast tissue, this protein helps cells divide normally. In certain cancers, however, CDK4/6 is no longer regulating, leaving cancer cells to multiply rapidly and uncontrollably.

CDK4/6 inhibitors may be part of your treatment for hormone-positive, HER2-negative metastatic breast cancers, or cancer with an overabundance of active hormone receptors, but not an overabundance of HER2. When combined with hormone therapy, these drugs may help keep cancer in check longer and improve response times.

mTOR inhibitors. These drugs may also be paired with hormone therapy in hormone receptor-positive, HER2-negative cancer. The drug interferes with *mTOR kinase,* a protein in your body that, if acting abnormally, can stimulate certain breast cancer growth. If these proteins are overactive, they even stop hormone therapy from working. When an mTOR inhibitor is added to your treatment plan, the treatment may resume working.

Poly (ADP-Ribose) polymerase inhibitors. If breast cancer cells become damaged, cellular proteins called *poly (ADP-ribose) polymerase (PARP)* helps them repair themselves. However, a *PARP inhibitor* prevents cancer cells from repairing themselves. For the small group of metastatic patients for whom PARP inhibitors are currently approved (those with BRCA1 and BRCA 2 mutations), the drugs can kill cancer cells. This may help keep the cancer in check.

PI3 kinase inhibitors. In 2019 a *PI3 kinase inhibitor* was approved for ER positive metastatic breast cancer, adding a new class of drug to treat this disease.

Chemotherapy

Even with increased use of hormone and other targeted drugs to slow metastatic breast cancer, chemotherapy is still a treatment option. The advantage is that it kills fast-growing cancer cells quickly, despite more toxic side effects than other therapies. For certain types of metastatic breast cancers, chemotherapy may be the only effective treatment.

If your cancer isn't fueled by either hormones or the HER2 proteins, chemotherapy is likely the best treatment option. It may also be a first choice if your cancer is spreading so quickly that you can't wait months for other drugs to take effect. Even if cancer responds to hormone therapy, for instance, your physician may order chemotherapy as a kick start. Chemotherapy may also be prescribed when hormone therapy no longer works. By disrupting the life cycle of cancer cells, chemotherapy offers an option for controlling the disease from spreading.

Follow-Up Care and Self-Care

As with primary breast cancer, regular monitoring of metastatic breast cancer is important. Keep follow-up medical appointments so that your physician can assess the status of your cancer and also any side effects related to treatment. Even though hormone therapy and other drugs are generally well tolerated, they still can cause digestive problems, pain, fatigue, and other issues.

Your physician's primary concern is how well your treatment is working. Has the cancer shrunk, grown, or stayed the same? Have you experienced any new symptoms? Your oncologist will be looking for signs that your cancer is stable, has improved, or has progressed.

What can you do to help yourself? As suggested earlier, eat nutritiously, exercise, control your weight, and avoid processed food and alcohol. Granted, there's no proof that after a cancer has spread these steps will change its course. Still, having a healthy lifestyle can help bolster your immune system so it will hopefully keep your cancer in check and prevent complications such as pneumonia. Make sure you have a source of emotional support.

As to long-term survival, statistics suggest that approximately 25 percent of stage IV breast cancer patients are alive at five years after diagnosis. Long-term success with treatment varies, depending on tumor characteristics and one's overall health.

Clinical Trials Offer Options

Should you join a clinical trial? Even though only 5 or 6 percent of cancer patients enroll in these trials, being open to the benefits of cancer research can be beneficial by giving you access to otherwise inaccessible tests and treatments. Breast cancer treatment is a rapidly changing field, but it's usually years before new therapies are FDA-approved and available. That includes options for treating metastatic disease. If you can undergo a promising drug or combined therapy still under study, your treatment may be more effective than standard treatment.

Your medical oncologist may already be participating in a clinical trial matching your diagnosis and treatment needs. If that's not the case, he or she likely knows of other studies for which you fit the screening criteria.

Before you commit, however, your physician will walk you through the details of a particular study, including possible side effects. If you do participate in a trial, your physician will still monitor your care.

Palliative Care

Specialized medical care for those with serious illness is called *palliative care*. The goal of this type of care is to improve quality of life of patients and their families. The focus is on relief for pain or other physical symptoms; this type of care is also intended to help with emotional concerns and family or spiritual issues. A patient may also seek help with goal setting and advance directives that specify what actions should be taken for their health care if they are no longer able to make decisions for themselves.

Any person living with a chronic illness, such as metastatic breast cancer, can benefit from the services of a palliative care provider. These services are often provided in the home or in an outpatient setting. Palliative care, along with appropriate treatments, helps individuals feel better and live longer.

In Good Company
(An inner dialogue)

"What do you mean, it was cancer?"

(I am too busy for that.)

"Yes, I'll be there in the morning."

(I don't mind losing a breast.)

"Please turn the morphine pump higher."

(Oh my God, this really hurts.)

"Your chemo will last only six months."

(Oh, well, a baby takes nine.)

"Is that a wig? You look stunning!"

(Surely he's flattering me.)

"Welcome: Breast Cancer Support Group."

(I am in good company.)

—*Suzanne W. Braddock, M.D.*

Resources

American Cancer Society (ACS)
15999 Clifton Road NE
Atlanta, GA 30329-4251
Phone: (800) ACS-2345 or (800) 227-2345
www.cancer.org

With more than two million volunteers and 3,400 local units, the ACS works to eliminate cancer as a major health problem through prevention, saving lives, and diminishing suffering through research, education, patient services, advocacy, and rehabilitation.

The ACS also sponsors "Look Good. Feel Better," a free, nonmedical, brand-neutral, national public service program created to help individuals with cancer look good, improve their self-esteem, and manage their treatment and recovery with greater confidence. Visit www.lookgoodfeelbetter.org.

The American Cancer Society also sponsors the Hope Lodge in many cities; each Hope Lodge offers cancer patients and their families a free, temporary place to stay when their best hope for effective treatment may be in another city. For more information, visit www.cancer.org/treatment/supportprogramsservices/hopelodge/index.

American Society of Breast Surgeons
10330 Old Columbia Road, Suite 100
Columbia, MD 21046
Phone: (410) 381-5470 or Toll free: (877) 992-5470
www.breastsurgeons.org
The American Society of Breast Surgeons Foundation is a charitable organization founded in 2005 dedicated to improving the standard of care for breast disease. It was established to support initiatives in the research and development of advanced breast disease treatments and technologies in order to improve the standards for superior patient care and education. They offer a state-of-the-art patient-access website for educational resources on breast disease awareness.

CHI Henry Lynch Cancer Center at Creighton University Medical Center Bergan Mercy
7500 Mercy Road
Omaha, NE 68124
Phone: (402) 717-2273
www.chihealth.com

Coping with Cancer Magazine
Phone: (615) 790-2400
www.copingmag.com/coping-with-cancer
A wide variety of professionals share their knowledge and experience in easy-to-read, relevant articles, and patients, caregivers, and survivors share their strategies for coping with cancer.

Food and Drug Administration (FDA)
10903 New Hampshire Avenue
Silver Spring, MD 20993
Phone: (888) INFO-FDA or (888) 463-6332
www.fda.gov
The Food and Drug Administration is a federal agency of the U.S. Department of Health and Human Services and is responsible for protecting and promoting public health through the regulation and supervision of food safety, tobacco prod-

ucts, dietary supplements, prescription and over-the-counter pharmaceutical drugs, vaccines, biopharmaceuticals, and other products.

Hereditary Cancer Center (HCC)

Creighton University
Department of Preventive Medicine
2500 California Plaza
Omaha, NE 68178
Phone: (402) 280-2700
https://medschool.creighton.edu/centers/hcc

The Hereditary Cancer Center (HCC) at Creighton University was established in 1984 in Omaha, Nebraska. The primary objective of the HCC is to conduct comprehensive research projects dealing with all types of cancer and is devoted to cancer prevention by identifying hereditary cancer syndromes. HCC conducts surveillance and management programs to oversee the natural history of these hereditary disorders.

MedlinePlus and PubMed Health

www.nlm.nih.gov/medlineplus
www.ncbi.nlm.nih.gov/pubmedhealth/

These two websites bring together authoritative information from the National Library of Medicine (NLM), the National Institutes of Health (NIH), and other government agencies and health-related organizations. Both sites provide easy access to medical journal articles and also have extensive information about drugs, an illustrated medical encyclopedia, interactive patient tutorials, and the latest health news.

National Cancer Institute (NCI)

National Institutes of Health
9000 Rockville Pike
Bethesda, MD 20892-2580
Phone: (301) 496-4000
(800) 4-CANCER or (800) 422-6237
www.cancer.gov

147

The NCI website offers recent cancer information from the National Cancer Institute, a component of the National Institutes of Health. Comprised of twenty-five separate institutes and centers, the NIH is one of eight health agencies in the U.S. Department of Health and Human Services.

National Coalition for Cancer Survivorship (NCCS)
8455 Colesville Road, Suite 930
Silver Spring, MD 20910
Phone: (877) NCCS-YES
www.canceradvocacy.org

Founded in 1986 by and for people with cancer and those who care for them, the National Coalition for Cancer Survivorship is a patient-led advocacy organization working on the behalf of people with all types of cancer and their families. Their mission is to ensure quality cancer care for all Americans by leading and strengthening the survivorship movement, empowering cancer survivors, and advocating for policy issues that affect cancer survivors' quality of life.

National Lymphedema Network, Inc.
411 Lafayette Street, 6th Floor
New York, NY 10003
Hotline: (800) 541-3259
Phone: (415) 908-3681
www.lymphnet.org

The mission of the NLN is to create awareness of lymphedema through education and to promote and support the availability of quality medical treatment for all individuals at risk for or affected by lymphedema. Their website offers community groups and discussions, research and article archives, and support for finding treatment of lymphedema.

GLOSSARY

A

accelerated partial breast irradiation (APBI): is radiation therapy delivered to only part of the breast over a period of days.

adjuvant therapy: anticancer drugs used in chemotherapy, hormone-blocking therapy, and targeted therapy, after surgery and/or radiation, to prevent recurrence or metastasis.

alkylators: a class of chemotherapy drugs that inhibit cell division and growth.

anastrozole: a drug used in hormone-blocking therapy.

anatomical implant: a breast implant that is fuller at the bottom than at the top; also called a *teardrop, contoured,* or *shaped implant.*

antimicrotubules: chemotherapy drugs that directly kill cancer cells with minimal damage to normal cells.

antineoplastics: chemotherapy drugs.

antitumor antibiotics: chemotherapy drugs.

areola: the darker-colored skin surrounding the nipple.

aromatase: an enzyme that converts other hormones to estrogen. It is the principal source of estrogen after menopause.

aromatase inhibitors: drugs that block estrogen production by inhibiting the hormone aromatase.

aspiration: a procedure in which a hollow needle withdraws fluid from a breast mass or other part of the body.

asymmetrical: having opposite sides or parts that do not precisely match, as when one breast is larger or smaller than the other.

axilla: armpit.

axillary dissection: surgical removal of lymph nodes in the armpit area.

axillary lymph nodes: group of twenty or more lymph nodes located in the deep tissues and around the armpit.

B

baseline: a condition against which later changes are compared, as in a baseline mammogram, usually taken before age forty.

benign: not cancerous.

bilateral: having two sides; affecting two sides equally, as in a bilateral mastectomy.

biopsy: a diagnostic procedure that removes tissue for microscopic analysis.

bisphosphonates: a class of drugs that disrupt the normal cycle in which bone breaks down and regenerates.

bone marrow: soft cell tissue in the bone center, where red blood cells, white blood cells, and platelets are manufactured.

bone-marrow aspiration: the withdrawal of bone marrow to be analyzed for the presence of free-floating cancer cells.

bone scan: a diagnostic test that detects areas of increased blood circulation in the bone.

boost treatments: tightly focused, additional doses of radiation, usually given for a week or two after standard radiation treatments have ended.

brachytherapy: radiation treatment delivered to a precise location by a device implanted inside the body.

BRCA1, BRCA2: genes, which, when mutated, are associated with hereditary breast cancer.

breast implant: a soft pouch, filled with saline or silicone, that is surgically implanted beneath the skin and muscle of the chest wall to form a reconstructed breast after mastectomy.

breast reconstruction: any surgical method used to create a new breast after mastectomy. The new breast will not produce milk and will not have sensation but will look like a normal breast.

Glossary

breast self-examination (BSE): a monthly routine in which a woman follows several steps to detect any changes or suspicious lumps in her breasts.

bulb: the smallest component in the milk-producing system of lobes in the breast.

C

cancer: a general term for diseases characterized by uncontrolled growth of abnormal cells that can invade and destroy healthy tissue. Also called *malignancy.*

capsular contracture: a complication following implant reconstruction in which scar tissue around the implant begins to contract and squeeze the implant.

carcinogen: a cancer-causing substance or agent.

carcinoma: the most common type of cancer, affecting skin, glands, or the lining of organs.

catheter: a tube-shaped medical device inserted into the body to keep a passage open or to facilitate the injection or withdrawal of fluids.

cell: the smallest structural unit of living tissue that can survive and reproduce on its own.

cell cycle: all cell activity from one cell division to the next.

chemotherapy: the administration of anticancer drugs that directly kill cancer cells or disrupt their ability to grow and reproduce.

clinical trial: a research project that tests drugs or other treatments on human subjects.

core biopsy: a diagnostic test in which a hollow needle removes small samples of tissue for laboratory analysis.

CT (computerized tomography) scan: a computer-aided method of creating three-dimensional images of organs and structures inside the body.

cyclophosphamide: an alkylator used in cancer treatment that attaches an alkyl group to DNA.

cytologist: a specialist who analyzes cells and diagnoses disease from cell abnormalities.

cytotoxic: toxic to cells; capable of destroying cells.

cyst: a benign, fluid-filled lump.

D

DCIS (ductal carcinoma *in situ*): a precancerous condition in which abnormal cells have been found in the milk ducts of the breast but have not broken through the duct walls.

density: thickness.

DES (diethylstilbestrol): a synthetic estrogen that was once prescribed to prevent complications in pregnancy; it is no longer used because it increases the risk of breast cancer.

diagnosis: the process of identifying a disease from its symptoms and from tests such as X-rays or biopsies; in breast cancer, determining the nature of a lump or any other change in the breast.

diagnostic mammogram: not a routine mammogram, but one ordered to investigate a lump found during breast self-examination (BSE) or a clinical examination.

DIEA (deep inferior epigastric artery) flap: a section of skin and fat moved up from the lower abdomen to the chest area and used for breast reconstruction after mastectomy.

diffuse: not localized in a single area.

digital mammography: a process in which the images produced on a mammogram machine are converted to computer code and then displayed in much finer detail than film can capture.

distant recurrence: a reappearance of cancer at a site other than the site of the original tumor.

DNA (deoxyribonucleic acid): the material that carries the genetic code, and establishes hereditary patterns, including inherited risks for certain diseases.

DNA repair enzyme inhibitors: chemotherapy drugs.

duct: a narrow tube that carries milk from the lobes of the breast to the nipple.

ductal carcinoma *in situ*: cancer that arises in the milk ducts.

ductal lavage: a diagnostic test in which a saline solution is introduced into the breast ducts and then withdrawn so that cells from the ducts can be analyzed for abnormalities.

Glossary

E

early detection: discovery of a cancer while it is still small—no more than two centimeters (less than an inch) in diameter—and before it has spread to lymph nodes near the breast.

enzyme: a complex protein that supports or initiates certain chemical reactions in the body.

epidermal growth factor receptor (EGFR): This cell-surface protein is a receptor for members of the epidermal growth factor family.

erythropoietin (EPO): a drug that stimulates the production of red blood cells.

estrogen: a female sex hormone produced by the ovaries, adrenal glands, placenta, and fatty tissues.

estrogen receptor: a location on a tumor at which estrogen molecules can attach; the presence of estrogen receptors means a tumor depends on estrogen to grow.

excisional biopsy: a surgical biopsy used for small tumors and capable of removing them completely.

exemestane: a drug used in hormone-blocking therapy; it blocks estrogen production in postmenopausal women by inhibiting the enzyme aromatase.

expander: a soft, empty pouch placed behind the chest muscle and gradually filled with saline over a period of months to stretch the skin before a breast implant is put in place.

external beam brachytherapy: a treatment that delivers radiation to a tumor area but requires no catheters or balloons.

external boost treatment: external beam radiation therapy delivered to a smaller area after a course of standard radiation therapy.

external radiation: radiation delivered from outside the body.

extrusion: the act of being forced through an opening, such as when an implant extrudes due to skin erosion.

F

false positive: a test that erroneously shows a positive result.

fibrocystic changes: a common condition in which the breasts develop benign, normal cysts that are sometimes mistaken for suspicious lumps. Often called *fibrocystic disease,* this condition is not actually an illness.

filgrastim: a drug that stimulates the production of red blood cells.

fine-needle aspiration (FNA): a kind of biopsy in which fluid is withdrawn (aspirated) using a fine, hollow needle. In the case of breast cancer, the fluid is aspirated from a tumor, and the cells within the fluid are examined for evidence of cancer.

G

genetic: having to do with the genes and hereditary characteristics.

gluteal flap: a wedge of skin, muscle, and fat taken from the buttocks to be used in breast reconstruction.

goserelin: a drug that suppresses estrogen production in premenopausal women.

graft: to surgically implant living tissue.

guided imagery: any of a number of techniques used to visualize images or imagine sensations in an effort to trigger a desired physical effect.

H

hematoma: a mass of blood that collects in tissue or organs. Breasts may be susceptible to hematomas after surgery.

Herceptin: a drug developed for women with HER2-positive breast cancer.

hereditary: genetically passed on by a parent or parents to offspring; the risk for some cancers is hereditary.

HER2/neu: a gene that helps control how cells grow, divide, and repair themselves, important in the control of abnormal or defective cells that could become cancerous.

hormone: a substance secreted by glands and circulated in the bloodstream to other parts of the body, where it exerts specific effects on cell activity.

hormone-blocking therapy: the use of drugs that block or disrupt the body's production of hormones in cases where a tumor depends on those hormones to grow.

hormone receptor: a location on a tumor at which either estrogen or progesterone molecules can attach; the presence of hormone receptors means a tumor depends on hormones to grow.

hyperplasia: uncontrolled, abnormally fast growth of cells.

hypofractionated radiation therapy: an accelerated course of radiation therapy, with higher doses given over the period of a few days.

I

image-guided biopsy: a technique in which computer images are used to guide a biopsy needle to a lump that cannot be felt but has shown up on a mammogram; also called a *stereotactic biopsy.*

immunohistochemical staining: a process in which living cells and tissues can be analyzed.

incisional biopsy: an open biopsy in which a small piece of a tumor is removed for laboratory analysis.

industry-based trials: a type of clinical trial sponsored by pharmaceutical companies in compliance with FDA requirements.

inflammatory breast cancer: a particularly aggressive form of breast cancer usually treated with chemotherapy before surgery.

infusion: slow drip of medication directly into a vein.

inhibitor: an agent used to reduce or slow the activity of a substance.

In situ: a term meaning "in position" or "in its place"; A breast cancer that has not spread through the wall of the milk duct or lobe where it originated is called *in situ.*

internal boost treatment: radiation therapy delivered internally to a small area after a course of standard radiation therapy.

invasive: cancer that is capable of invading, or has invaded, breast tissue beyond the wall of the duct or lobe in which it has arisen.

K

Ki-67: a protein whose growth rate in cancer cells can be measured to help determine how fast a tumor is growing.

L

lactation: milk production in the breast.

lapatinib: a drug used as a targeted breast cancer therapy.

latissimus dorsi flap: a section of muscle, skin, and some fat taken from the latissimus dorsi muscle of the upper back and used to form a new breast after mastectomy.

LCIS (lobular carcinoma *in situ*): the presence of abnormal cells within a lobe or lobes of one or both breasts; the cells have not spread beyond the walls of any lobes. The presence of LCIS indicates a heightened risk for either invasive lobular or ductal cancer.

letrazole: a drug used in hormone-blocking therapy; it blocks estrogen production in postmenopausal women by inhibiting the enzyme aromatase.

linear accelerator: the machine most commonly used to deliver radiation treatments.

lobe: one of fifteen to twenty rounded divisions in each breast; the part of the breast in which milk is produced.

lobular carcinoma: cancer that originates in the milk-producing lobules of the breast.

lobule: one of several small components of a lobe.

local cancer: cancer that is occurring in only one part of the body.

local recurrence: reappearance of cancer at the site of the original tumor.

local treatment: treatment of cancer at the site of the tumor by surgery or radiation.

lumpectomy: breast cancer surgery that removes only the tumor and a surrounding margin of healthy tissue to be examined for cancer cells; also called a *wide excision* or *partial mastectomy.*

lymph, lymphatic fluid: a clear, yellowish fluid containing white blood cells that bathes body tissues and carries waste products away through lymph vessels.

lymphedema: a persistent swelling caused by excess fluid that may collect when the lymph nodes and vessels are removed. This condition can occur at any time after surgery, including years later.

lymph nodes: small masses of lymphatic tissue distributed along the lymph vessels and containing lymphocytes that filter waste products from lymphatic fluid.

lymph vessels: similar to blood vessels but with the purpose of circulating lymphatic fluid through the body and to the lymph nodes.

M

magnetic resonance imaging (MRI): a diagnostic imaging test that uses a powerful magnet and radio waves to show differences in the number of blood vessels in various types of body tissue. Cancerous tissue tends to have more blood vessels than healthy tissue.

malignant: cancerous.

MammaPrint: molecular diagnostic test that is used to assess the risk that a breast tumor will spread to other parts of the body.

mammogram: an image of the breast created by mammography.

mammography: the use of X-rays to examine the breasts for tumors or microcalcifications.

Mammotome: a biopsy that uses suction and a large tube to withdraw breast tissue; also called *vacuum-assisted biopsy.*

margin: healthy tissue surrounding a tumor, removed at the same time as the tumor for laboratory analysis.

marker: a mechanism that identifies, characterizes, or predicts.

mastectomy: surgical removal of the breast.

mastitis: infection of the breast.

medical oncologist: a physician who specializes in systemic cancer treatments.

menopause: the permanent cessation of menstrual periods, usually in a woman's late forties to early fifties.

metachronous: occurring in a series.

metastasis: the spread of cancer from its original site to another part of the body or lymphatic system.

metastasizing: spreading to other parts of the body.

metastatic breast cancer: breast cancer that has spread beyond the breast and nearby lymph nodes to a distant part of your body.

microcalcifications: tiny, grain-sized deposits of calcium in breast tissue, detectable by mammogram; when they appear in clusters, they are a sign of DCIS.

microcatheter: an extremely small tube used in ductal lavage.

micrometastasis: the early spread of cancer from the original tumor by means of random, microscopic cancer cells that have not yet formed a mass and are generally not detectable. (However, bone-marrow aspiration can detect micrometastases when the cancer has begun to spread to bone.)

microtubule: very small tubules within the cytoplasm of a cell.

microtubule inhibitor: a chemotherapy drug.

modified radical mastectomy: surgery that removes the entire breast and the axillary lymph nodes.

monoclonal antibody: an antibody derived from a single cell to act against a certain antigen.

multifocal: having more than one location. A multifocal breast cancer is present simultaneously in more than one lobe or duct.

mutation: a change in a cell's DNA.

myocutaneous: comprising muscle, skin, and fat. A myocutaneous flap is taken from one part of the body to reconstruct another, such as a surgically removed breast.

N

negative biopsy: a biopsy in which no cancer cells are seen in the tissue or fluid removed.

neoadjuvant therapy: chemotherapy or hormone-blocking therapy given before surgery to shrink a tumor to operable size.

neoplasia: the process in which a tumor forms.

nipple: the portion of the breast that protrudes and through which milk is drawn.

nipple-areola: the nipple and surrounding shaded area.

node-negative: showing no evidence of cancer in the lymph nodes. A breast tumor is deemed node-negative when axillary dissection or sentinel node biopsy finds no cancer cells.

non-opioid: non-narcotic medication.

O

oncogene: a mutated gene associated with a heightened risk of cancer.

oncologist: a medical doctor who specializes in cancer treatment.

Oncotype DX: a diagnostic test that quantifies the likelihood of disease recurrence in women with early-stage breast cancer.

open biopsy: any surgical biopsy.

opioid: narcotic medication.

osteoporosis: a disease in which the bones become more porous and more susceptible to breakage as a person ages.

P

pamidronate: one of a class of drugs called *bisphosphonates,* which have been shown in some studies to prevent the spread of breast cancer to bone or to treat the cancer effectively if it does spread.

pathologist: a medical specialist who analyzes biopsied tissue under a microscope and diagnoses disease from any abnormalities that are present.

pathology report: the pathologist's written record of the analysis of biopsied tissue.

patient-controlled analgesia (PCA): is a method of pain control that gives patients the power to control their pain. With PCA, a computerized pump contains a syringe of pain medication as prescribed by a doctor, is connected directly to a patient's intravenous (IV) line.

peau d'orange: skin texture like that of an orange; a symptom of inflammatory breast cancer.

pectoralis minor: a small, strap-like muscle running from the outer edge of the collarbone to the top of the breast, sometimes removed during axillary dissection.

pegfilgrastim: a drug given in conjunction with chemotherapy to lessen its toxic effects.

p53 gene: a gene that normally acts as a tumor suppressor but when abnormal, may be associated with a high risk of breast cancer.

phantom breast: the sensation that a surgically removed breast is still present.

plant alkaloids: chemotherapy drugs.

plastic surgeon: a specialist in cosmetic and reconstructive surgery.

platelets: blood cells that aid clotting.

polygenic breast cancer: cancer that usually shows up in more than one member of an extended family.

port: a small, semipermanent opening that is surgically implanted just under the skin. It is attached to a tube leading directly to a large vein. A port may be used when repeated injections are necessary, since it eliminates the need to tap a new vein each time.

positron emission tomography (PET) scan: a diagnostic imaging test that reveals cell activity by detecting the different rates at which different cells consume sugar or glucose. Cancer cells consume glucose more rapidly than normal cells.

postmenopausal: after menopause.

preinvasive: malignant cells that are capable of becoming invasive but have yet to spread into surrounding tissues.

premenopausal: before menopause.

primary cancer: a first-occurring tumor.

progesterone: a female sex hormone produced by the ovaries.

progesterone receptor: a location on a tumor at which progesterone molecules can attach.

progestin: synthetic progesterone.

prognosis: the likely outcome of a disease; in the case of breast cancer, the statistical chance of long-term, disease-free survival.

prophylactic: preventive. A prophylactic mastectomy is performed when no cancer is present but the risk of breast cancer is high.

prosthesis: an external breast form worn by some women after mastectomy.

protocol: a document listing all steps, procedures, safety measures, and research methods to be used in a clinical trial.

Q

quadrant: any of the four segments into which a body part can be divided vertically and horizontally.

quadrantectomy: a partial mastectomy involving removal of the quadrant of the breast in which the tumor is located.

quality-of-life trials: a type of clinical trial that focuses on issues such as pain management and chronic side effects.

R

radiation oncologist: a medical doctor who specializes in radiation therapy.

radiation pneumonitis: a short-term inflammation of lung tissue caused by exposure to radiation therapy.

radiation therapy: a local treatment in which a radioactive beam is used to kill cancer cells in the area of the tumor.

radical mastectomy: an invasive surgical procedure that removes the breast, the axillary lymph nodes, and the muscle of the chest wall. Radical mastectomy is almost never used today.

radiologist: a medical doctor who specializes in the interpretation of X-ray images for diagnosis.

raloxifene: one of the class of drugs called *SERMs,* used in hormone-blocking therapy.

receptors: a cell or a group of cells to which the hormones estrogen and progesterone can attach themselves.

reconstructive surgery: the use of plastic surgery to model a new breast after mastectomy, using either breast implants or tissue from elsewhere in the body. The reconstructed breast looks like a normal breast but is not functional and does not have sensation.

recurrence: the reappearance of cancer after an initial course of treatment has ended; recurrence can be local or distant.

red blood cells: cells that carry oxygen, which gives the body fuel for energy.

retraction: a drawing-in or drawing-back. When the nipple or the skin of the breast retracts, it can be a sign of inflammatory breast cancer.

S

saline: a sterile, saltwater solution.

screening mammogram: a routine mammogram usually performed annually to check for indications of breast cancer.

sentinel node: the first lymph node to which lymphatic fluid drains from the area of a tumor; therefore, the first in which spreading cancer cells are likely to show up.

sentinel node biopsy: a procedure that removes a sample of tissue from the sentinel node for examination under a microscope. If the sentinel node is free of cancer, the other nodes do not need to be removed and examined, and surgery is minimized.

sentinel node mapping: locating the sentinel node.

SERM (selective estrogen receptor modulator): one of a category of drugs that block either hormone production in the body or the hormone receptors on tumors, thus depriving certain cancers of the hormones they need for growth.

side effect: an undesirable effect of surgery, chemotherapy, radiation, or other treatment. Some side effects include pain, nausea, skin changes, hair loss, or fatigue.

silicone: a synthetic material used to encase and fill some breast implants.

simple bilateral mastectomy: the surgical removal of all breast tissue from both breasts with no removal of lymph nodes; also called *total bilateral mastectomy*.

simple mastectomy: the surgical removal of all breast tissue but no lymph nodes; also called *total mastectomy*.

spiculated: star-shaped; a spiculated mass on a mammogram that should be biopsied for cancer cells.

spiral CT scan: a CT scan in which the X-ray beam rotates around you in a spiral; also called *helical CT scan*.

sporadic breast cancer: breast cancer in a patient with no known family history of the disease.

stage: the grading system for the severity of a disease.

stage migration: when breast cancer is identified as being at a different stage in its development due to new breast cancer staging guidelines.

stem cell rescue: drugs given to stimulate the production of bone-marrow stem cells.

stem cell transplant: a procedure for regenerating bone marrow destroyed by high doses of chemotherapy drugs. Bone-marrow stem cells (cells capable of forming blood cells) are removed before chemotherapy and then reintroduced afterward to restore bone marrow and its production of blood cells.

Glossary

stereotactic biopsy: a technique in which computer images are used to guide a biopsy needle to a lump that cannot be felt but has shown up on a mammogram; also called *image-guided biopsy.*

submuscular: the placement of a breast implant beneath the pectoral muscle.

surgical biopsy: using an incision for the removal of part or all of a lump or suspicious area to be examined by a pathologist; also called *open biopsy.*

symmetry shapers: products that can be placed in a bra to achieve a symmetrical appearance post-mastectomy; also called *balance shapers.*

synchronous: occurring at the same time.

systemic treatment: a cancer treatment such as chemotherapy that travels throughout the body to destroy random, microscopic cancer cells that may have spread beyond the site of the original tumor.

T

tamoxifen: an estrogen-blocking drug used in treating and preventing breast cancer.

targeted therapy: administration of a drug created to target cancer cells.

taxane: one of several chemotherapy drugs that directly kill cancer cells with minimal damage to healthy cells.

temporary radiation implants: small catheters used to deliver radiation.

Three-D mammogram: also referred to as *digital breast tomosynthesis.* A screening test that creates three-dimensional pictures of the breast with X-rays.

tissue expander: a temporary balloon-like device, made of elastic silicone rubber, used to stretch the skin in the breast area following mastectomy.

tissue expansion: a process in which a soft, empty pouch is placed behind the chest muscle and gradually filled with saline over a period of months; this stretches the skin to accommodate a breast implant.

tomosynthesis: an FDA-approved, digital screening test for breast cancer. Also referred to as *3-D mammography,* it provides a clearer picture of breast tissues than a regular mammogram.

topoisomerase inhibitor: a chemotherapy drug.

total mastectomy: the surgical removal of all breast tissue but no lymph nodes; also called *simple mastectomy.*

toxic: poisonous.

TRAM flap: a section of muscle, skin, and fat moved up from the lower abdomen to the chest area and used for breast reconstruction after mastectomy.

transducer: a microphone-like device that's passed over the skin during an ultrasound test.

trastuzumab: a monoclonal antibody used to treat breast cancer

tumor: an abnormal growth of cells or tissue. Tumors can be benign (noncancerous) or malignant (cancerous).

tyrosine kinase inhibitor: a drug used in targeted therapy.

U

ultrasonography: the use of high-frequency sound waves to generate images of internal organs or tumors. Ultrasonography can determine whether a suspicious lump is filled with fluid or is solid; if it is solid, it could be cancerous and should be tested further.

V

vascular: of or relating to blood vessels.

visualization: the formation of visual images.

W

white blood cells: cells that fight infection.

wide excision: removal of a breast tumor and surrounding margin of normal tissue; also called a *lumpectomy.*

INDEX

Index

Index

Index

Index

vaginal dryness, 116, 119
visualization, 43
vitamins, 44, 109

W

warning signs of breast cancer,
    11, 14, 124
    during BSE, 13
weight gain, 44, 113, 114, 116,
    119
weight loss, 113
well-differentiated breast cancer
    cells, 30, 123
white blood cells, 3, 68, 113
wigs and hairpieces, 115
William Beaumont Hospital, 105
women's health groups, 56

X

X-rays, 5, 15, 17, 20, 103, 127,
    135

Y

yoga, 43, 44

ABOUT THE AUTHORS

Suzanne W. Braddock, M.D., has been a breast cancer survivor since 1992. She is a retired dermatologist in Omaha, Nebraska. Born and raised in New Jersey, Dr. Braddock received her medical training at the Medical College of Pennsylvania, Philadelphia, and at the University of Nebraska Medical School, Omaha. Dr. Braddock is the author of several scientific publications. She has a daughter, Gail.

Jane M. Kercher, M.D., F.A.C.S., is a general and oncological surgeon in Denver, Colorado. She received her medical training at the University of Utah Medical School, Salt Lake City, and at the University of Nebraska Medical School, Omaha, Nebraska. Dr. Kercher is an associate professor of surgery at the Colorado School of Medicine, Denver, Colorado, and was also an associate professor of surgery at the University of Nebraska Medical School prior to her move to Colorado.

Dr. Kercher remains active in educational presentations. She serves on several local and state cancer committees, and is chair of the Breast Program Leadership at the Invision Sally Jobe Breast Program, Englewood, Colorado. A native of Wyoming, Dr. Kercher lives in Denver. Her son Matthew is neurosurgical resident at the University of California, Davis, Sacramento, California.

John J. Edney, M.D., F.A.C.S., a plastic surgeon in private practice in Omaha, Nebraska, specializes in postmastectomy breast reconstruction and cosmetic surgery. Dr. Edney is the chief of the Division of Plastic Surgery at the Nebraska Methodist Hospital. He is an assistant clinical professor of surgery at the University of Nebraska Medical School, Omaha, and Creighton University School of Medicine. Dr. Edney and his wife, Pat, have three children—Christopher, Matthew, and Jennifer.

Margaret Block, M.D., F.A.C.P., is a medical oncologist with Nebraska Cancer Specialists in Omaha, Nebraska. Board-certified in both internal medicine and medical oncology, Dr. Block treats many women with breast cancer. She is a native of New York City and attended Albany Medical College in Albany, New York; she received her medical oncology training at the University of Wisconsin in Madison, Wisconsin. Dr. Block is a member of the U.S. Oncology Breast Cancer Committee. She also serves on several local breast cancer boards.

Melanie Morrissey Clark has been a professional writer and editor for more than thirty years. Ms. Clark is president of Clark Creative Group in Omaha. She holds a bachelor of science degree in journalism from the University of Nebraska. She lives in Omaha with her husband, Fred Clark, and their triplets, Cooper, Sophie, and Simon.

Consumer Health Titles from Addicus Books

Visit our online catalog at www.AddicusBooks.com

To Order Books:
Visit us online at: www.AddicusBooks.com
Call toll free: (800) 888-4741

For discounts on bulk purchases,
call our Special Sales Department at (402) 330-7493,
or e-mail us at *info@Addicus Books.com*

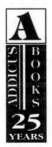

Addicus Books
P. O. Box 45327
Omaha, NE 68145

*Addicus Books is dedicated to publishing consumer health books
that comfort and educate.*

New Editions of Our Best-Selling Oncology Books

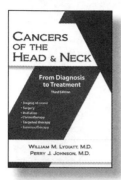

CANCERS OF THE HEAD AND NECK
From Diagnosis to Treatment
Third Edition
William M. Lydiatt, M.D.
Perry J. Johnson, M.D.
ISBN: 9781943886821
190 pages • trade paper
$19.95 • February 2019

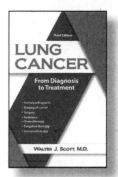

LUNG CANCER
From Diagnosis to Treatment
Third Edition
Walter J. Scott, M.D.
ISBN: 9781943886678
140 pages • trade paper
$19.95 • January 2019

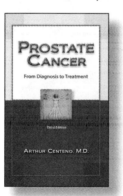

PROSTATE CANCER
From Diagnosis to Treatment
Third Edition
Arthur Centeno, M.D.
ISBN: 9781943886845
128 pages • trade paper
$19.95 • January 2019

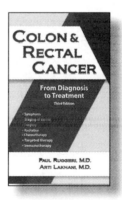

COLON & RECTAL CANCER
From Diagnosis to Treatment
Third Edition
Paul Ruggieri, M.D.
Arti Lakhani, M.D.
ISBN: 9781943886838
158 pages • trade paper
$19.95 • March 2019

Addicus Books health titles include:
Index • Glossary • Illustrations • Photos • Resource Section